The Meditative Path to Health

Harnessing the Mind-Body Connection

Dr. Manmohan Chaturvedi

Dedication

This book is dedicated to my spiritual Guru Shri Vethathiri Maharishi*. The seeds of spirituality sown by His divine self during my formative years have guided me on this journey and by His blessings now I feel ready to share with others the insights gained in this process.

* Shri Vethathiri Maharishi (1911–2006) was a spiritual leader and founder-trustee of 'The World Community Service Centre'. Link to his biodata is given below:
https://www.vethathiri.edu.in/pages/vethathiri-maharishi

Table of Contents

Contents	Content's heading	Page Number
Dedication		IV
Table of Contents		V
Foreword		VIII
About the Author		XI
Preface		XII
PART I	FOUNDATIONS	1
Chapter 1	Consciousness and Cosmos	3
Chapter 2	The Science of Self-Healing	14
Chapter 3	Understanding Your Inner Biology	27
Chapter 4	The Power of Meditation	40
PART II	THE MIND AS MEDICINE	52
Chapter 5	Breaking the Addiction to the Past	53
Chapter 6	Cultivating Positive Expectancy	63
Chapter 7	Stress, Telomeres, and the Meditative Solution	73
PART III	THE PRACTICE	86
Chapter 8	Meditation for Genetic Expression	87
Chapter 9	The Emotional Connection	98
Chapter 10	Living in the Quantum Field	105
PART IV	PHILOSOPHY OF MEDITATION	110
Chapter 11	Patanjali Yoga Sutra	111
Chapter 12	Integration of Patanjali Yoga Sutra in Daily Life	123

Appendix 'A'	Comprehensive Cellular Biology Glossary	137
Appendix 'B'	Comprehensive Meditation Practice Glossary	149
Bibliography	Chapter wise relevant references are listed here for a deep dive by interested reader	172
Index	Alphabetic index of important topics with page numbers	182

Foreword

This book by Dr. Chaturvedi attempts to explore the intersection of two revolutionary scientific perspectives: the placebo effect as a demonstration of the mind's healing capacity, and telomere biology as a measurable indicator of cellular ageing and renewal. By weaving these concepts together through the practice of meditation, he delineates a pathway to not just manage stress or find momentary peace, but potentially influence the very mechanisms that determine how our cells age and regenerate.

Meditation serves as a perfect bridge between the placebo effect and telomere biology because the mind-body connection has been known to researchers for a long time and meditation is a known technique to influence mind in a deliberate manner.

When we integrate these scientific perspectives, a new paradigm emerges: the mind as medicine. This isn't merely positive thinking or wishful visualization. Rather, it's the recognition that consciousness itself may be a biological force—one that can influence gene expression, modulate immune function, regulate stress responses, and potentially even affect how our cells age.

This perspective doesn't diminish the value of conventional medical treatments. Instead, it suggests that our internal mental environment creates a biological context that can either amplify or diminish the effectiveness of any intervention, whether pharmaceutical, surgical, or lifestyle-based.

The value of this book lies in suggesting meditation as a way of life to help us maintain a good physical and mental health using the emerging research findings in biology and psychiatry.

I wish this book a success in helping the reader towards a healthy and long life by adopting simple to practice lifestyle changes.

Dr. Alok Pandey, MD (Psychiatry)*

*Dr. Alok Pandey is a medical doctor, specifically a psychiatrist, based in Pondicherry. He is a well-known figure associated with the Sri Aurobindo Ashram. He has a strong interest in Sri Aurobindo and the Mother's teachings, particularly in the fields of yoga, psychology, education, and health.

About the Author

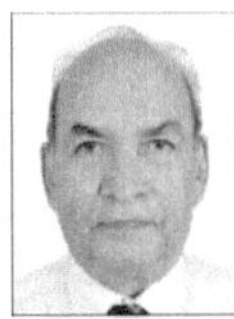

Dr Manmohan Chaturvedi is an engineer by profession and holds a PhD. from IIT Delhi. He served the Indian Air Force for about 35 years and retired from the rank of Air Commodore.

He has published few books on spirituality and technology and details of these books are available at link below:

https://notionpress.com/author/1039052?srsltid=AfmBOorp3r1 2RqNVs2btNsJQXZMwBIH-yOijfxOpjC02cNMltqo1znzw

He had interest in Spirituality since college days and was formally initiated in meditation by Shri Vethathiri Maharishi in 1982. With a purpose to share understanding gathered while reading scriptures and books on philosophy, he is regularly sharing his insights in a Spiritual blog.

Link to the blog 'Search within' is shared below: https://search-within-self.blogspot.com/

Preface

To attempt a book on such esoteric theme as, 'using Meditation for Health', is strange for a person with no real knowledge of human biology.

This theme attracted my attention few months ago after I read a book title ' You Are the Placebo: Making Your Mind Matter' by Joe Dispenza. However,the real trigger came in the form of another interesting book 'The Telomere Effect: A Revolutionary Approach to Living Younger, Healthier, Longer' by Elizabeth Blackburn, Elissa Epel.

Both books have explored, besides other things , positive effect of meditation in improving our cellular health and help us live longer with disease free old age.Treatment of physical ailments using effect of mind over body is also explored by the first book.

High readability of both these books has primarily helped me to understand the scientific facts enumerated in them. I got emboldened by this fact and my familiarity with meditation and experiencing positive effects on my body and mind was additional reason for me to toy with the idea of putting meditative practices as the third element in exploring a mix with the key ideas elaborated in these two books.

Thus, I have attempted a short book in simple language towards helping readers like me, with little specialised knowledge, to apply the key ideas elaborated in the two books through lens of meditative practices in achieving healthy living.

However, the key theme of this book i.e. meditative practices is possible only if the reader has some idea of one's true self.

Normally, we associate with our body and mind apparatus as our true self and this may lead to a challenge while attempting meditation as a tool for conscious attempts towards achieving healthy living, both at mental or physical level.

This process of creating a gap between our consciousness and body-mind apparatus is not a trivial task. Meditation is a technique to put us in contact with our true self. Only when we are operating from our true self can we hope to consciously intervene on our thoughts and cellular biology of our physical body. Modern research, based on empirical evidence, as brought out by the two books referred above is only pointing out to this deep and inevitable connection of our consciousness or true self to the processes at our mental and physical level.

Thus, in writing this book I am trying to borrow credibility from contemporary research for an ancient Hindu thought governing all our worldly experiences. Wihout understanding this connect of our true self with the body and mind , all meditative practices and positive suggestions to intervene at the physical and mental level would be futile.

Contemporary research confirms the mind-body connection, aligning with ancient Hindu wisdom that emphasizes the interconnectedness of mind, body, and spirit. Modern science explores the physiological mechanisms, while ancient texts like the Patanjali Yoga Sutras and Ayurvedic principles provide frameworks for understanding and managing this relationship for holistic well-being[1].

---

[1] Shamasundar C. *Relevance of ancient Indian wisdom to modern mental health - A few examples. Indian J Psychiatry. 2008 Apr;50(2):138-43. doi: 10.4103/0019-5545.42404. PMID: 19742213; PMCID: PMC2738332.*

In Bhagwad Gita chapter 13, Lord Krishna shares this eternal secret of our existence with his disciple Arjuna.The chapter introduces two fundamental concepts: the "field" (our body and material world) and the "knower of the field" (our soul/consciousness that observes everything). Think of it like a movie - there's the movie screen (field) and the person watching the movie (knower)[2].

The "field" represents the physical body and the material world, composed of the five elements and undergoes changes. This includes:

- Our physical body
- Our mind and emotions
- Our environment
- Everything we can see, touch, or experience

The "knower of the field" refers to the soul, the conscious observer within that remains unchanging and eternal.This is:

- Our true self/consciousness
- The witness that observes all your experiences
- The part of us that never changes despite bodily changes

Without clarity on above concepts and deep faith in its universal application, our positive suggestions through our thoughts would lack the conviction and our motivation may sag.

---

[2] *https://www.thedivineindia.com/bhagavad-gita-chapter-13-the-illuminating-path-of-knowledge/7331*

This book is meant to be an experiential guide based on the eternal principle of Hindu thought and the current scientific research evidence.

Our meditation practices would certainly help us achieve desired positive results and at the same time bring us closer to our true self. Knowing the principle behind is just a good beginning but practice of this meditative approach would only get us the desired results over time. No miracle is promised.

Now, I welcome you to a journey into the fascinating intersection of mind, body, and cellular health. This book explores the revolutionary idea that our thoughts, emotions, and beliefs have a direct and profound impact on our physical well-being, particularly at the cellular level.

We will delve into the science behind this connection, drawing from groundbreaking research on telomeres, the protective caps at the end of our chromosomes, and the powerful phenomenon called 'Placebo effect'.

Our aim is not merely to present scientific facts in simple language but to provide a practical guide to harness the innate healing potential within each of us.

We will explore the ancient wisdom of meditation and mindfulness practices, combined with modern scientific understanding, to unlock pathways for cellular renewal and transformation to our ageing bodies and our stressed out minds. We will discover how chronic stress can accelerate ageing at the cellular level and how skillfully managing stress through specific meditative techniques can reverse this process. We will delve into the biochemistry of emotions and how our habitual emotional states influence our biological environment.

Through detailed instructions and protocols, we will learn various meditation practices designed to optimize genetic expression, cultivate positive expectancy, and thus break free from our limiting patterns that are rooted in our past.

Considering the pivotal role of Consciousness to our discourse in this book and its interaction with our body-mind apparatus and the world surrounding us we have elaborated on this crucial topic in chapter 1 titled ' Consciousness and Cosmos' in this book. Knowledge of the consciousness is crucial to view this world in a pragmatic manner and face the tribulations of life with equanimity.

Philosophical basis of meditation is explained through a discourse of Patanjali's Yoga Sutra in chapter 11 followed by suggestions for integrating these principles in our daily life in concluding chapter 12.

Each chapter builds upon the previous, providing a comprehensive roadmap to understanding and applying these powerful principles. Whether you are new to meditation or an experienced practitioner, this book offers insights and practical techniques to enhance your well-being and deepen your understanding of the profound mind-body connection.

My hope is that this book empowers you to take an active role in your health and healing journey, transforming not only your physical well-being but also your consciousness and experience of life. Prepare to embark on a transformative journey that will unlock the extraordinary potential within you.

In compiling this book, I have extensively used internet resources and AI tools to help me organize the text on various facets of current research in the domains that this book addresses.

Thus, an attempt is made to ensure that salient and topical texts in relevant domains of our interest are adequately covered. My experience and insights helped me to validate and improve the contents further.
At appendices 'A' and 'B' exhaustive glossaries on 'Cellular Biology' and 'Meditation Practice' have been provided for helping the reader with specialised terms of two domains that constitute the core of this book.

Manmohan Chaturvedi

PART I

FOUNDATIONS

1. Consciousness and the Cosmos

Introduction: The Enigma of Consciousness
This chapter attempts to describe the concept of human Consciousness from both ancient Hindu perspective and ongoing modern sciencetific research. The relationship of this Consciousness with the Cosmos around us is to be understood before we can possibly use meditative approaches towards a healthy life.

Consciousness, the subjective experience of being aware, stands as one of the most profound mysteries in our understanding of reality. It is the lens through which we perceive the universe, yet its nature and relationship to the physical world remain deeply puzzling.

In modern science, consciousness has emerged as a frontier of inquiry, challenging our understanding of the brain, mind, and the nature of reality itself. From the role of the observer in quantum mechanics to the hard problem of consciousness in philosophy of mind, questions about awareness and experience permeate cutting-edge research.

In Hindu philosophy, particularly in schools like Advaita Vedanta, consciousness (often termed Chit) is not merely a product of material processes but is considered fundamental to the nature of reality.

In this chapter, we will delve into the nature of consciousness from both scientific and Hindu philosophical perspectives. We will explore how these different approaches conceptualize consciousness, its relationship to the physical world, and its potential role in the cosmos at large. By examining these questions through multiple lenses, we aim to develop a richer, more nuanced understanding of consciousness and its place in our conception of cosmos.

Scientific Perspectives on Consciousness

The scientific study of consciousness has gained significant momentum in recent decades, drawing insights from neuroscience, psychology, physics, and philosophy. Let's explore key aspects of the scientific approach to consciousness:

Neuroscientific Approaches

Neuroscience seeks to understand consciousness by studying the brain and nervous system:

- Neural Correlates of Consciousness (NCCs): Identifying brain activity patterns associated with conscious experiences.
- Global Workspace Theory: Proposes that consciousness arises from the global broadcast of information in the brain.
- Integrated Information Theory: Suggests that consciousness is intrinsic to certain physical systems and can be quantified.

Cognitive and Psychological Approaches

Cognitive science and psychology examine consciousness through mental processes and behavior:

- Attention and Awareness: Studying the relationship between attention mechanisms and conscious perception.
- Unconscious Processing: Exploring the vast realm of mental processes that occur outside of awareness.
- Altered States of Consciousness: Investigating experiences like meditation, psychedelic states, and near-death experiences.

Quantum Approaches to Consciousness

Some researchers have proposed that quantum mechanics may play a role in consciousness:

- Orchestrated Objective Reduction (Orch-OR): Penrose and Hameroff's theory suggesting quantum processes in microtubules give rise to consciousness.
- Quantum Mind Theories: Various proposals that quantum effects in the brain could explain features of consciousness like free will or non-locality.

Philosophical Approaches

Philosophy of mind grapples with fundamental questions about the nature of consciousness:

- **The Hard Problem of Consciousness**: David Chalmers' formulation of the challenge of explaining why we have subjective experiences.
- **Dualism vs. Materialism**: Debates about whether consciousness is separate from or emergent from physical processes.
- **Panpsychism**: The view that consciousness is a fundamental feature of the universe, present to some degree in all matter.

Artificial Intelligence and Consciousness

The development of AI raises new questions about the nature of consciousness:

- Can machines be conscious? What would be required for artificial consciousness?
- The Chinese Room Argument[3] and other challenges to machine consciousness.

The Chinese Room Argument, a thought experiment proposed by John Searle, argues that a computer's ability to perform complex tasks, such as translating Chinese, does not equate to genuine understanding or intelligence. It challenges the idea of strong AI,

---

[3] *https://plato.stanford.edu/entries/chinese-room/*

which posits that computers can have minds with the same level of understanding as humans.

- Implications of potential artificial consciousness for our understanding of mind and reality.

Consciousness in Hindu Philosophy

Hindu philosophy, particularly in its Vedantic forms, places consciousness at the center of its understanding of reality.

Vedanta accepts five means of knowledge, namely, Pratyaksha, Anuman, Upamana, Arthapatti and Shastra or Shabda. The explanation of these is given below:

- Pratyaksha: Perception, or direct sensory experience

- Anumana: Inference, or reasoning based on perception

- Upamana: Comparison, or analogy

- Arthapatti: Presumption, or postulation to explain unobservable phenomena

- Shastra/Shabda: Verbal testimony, or credible sources

The first four are used to gain knowledge of the world as we perceive. The last means is to know Brahman.

The first four depend on perception (pratyaksha) as the basic means. Perception has the limitations of the perceiver, the instruments and the perceived object. Thus it cannot give any holistic knowledge.

Hence even science which uses these four means always finds a limit to whatever they understand. They always arrive at some subtle effect rather than the ultimate cause of the world.

Shastra (Scriptures) praman (means of knowledge) which is Anadi (without beginning), Ananta (endless) and Apaurusheya (not of a man) alone remains the means to know about the ultimate cause of this world and its nature.

The knowledge happens in Buddhi (Intellect). When we use the above four means to know the world the appropriate thoughts takes place in the buddhi which we call knowledge.

When we use the Shastra (Scriptures) as means to know Brahman, it uses the technique of neti neti (negation- not this not this). When all the qualities of world are negated what remains in the buddhi is an image of Brahman. Like in a mirror when all objects are negated what remains is an image of space. This image is called Akhandakar vritti (constant awareness). Akhandakara vritti is a concept in Vedanta that describes the constant awareness of being the light of consciousness in every objective knowledge. It means that even though the vrittis of objects are broken, there is a continuous flow of thoughts and reflection of the light of consciousness.

This is a theoretical understanding of Brahman. Shastra says this Brahman is not different from our own self which is experienced as thoughtless 'I' (as in deep sleep). To constantly assert this Brahman as our self is the practice is nididhyasana (vedantic meditation) which ultimately culminates in experience which is called Aparokshanubuti (self realisation).

Let's explore key concepts related to consciousness in Hindu thought:

Atman and Brahman

- **Atman**: The individual self or consciousness, often considered identical with Brahman.

- **Brahman**: The ultimate reality, often described as pure consciousness (Chit).

- **The Mahavakya "Tat Tvam Asi" (That Thou Art)**: Expressing the identity of individual consciousness with universal consciousness.

Levels of Consciousness

Many Hindu texts describe different states or levels of consciousness:

- **Waking (Jagrat)**: Ordinary waking consciousness.
- **Dreaming (Swapna)**: The consciousness experienced in dreams.
- **Deep Sleep (Sushupti)**: A state of potential consciousness without objects.
- **Turiya**: The fourth state, transcending the other three, often equated with pure consciousness.

Consciousness as Fundamental

- In Advaita Vedanta, consciousness is not an emergent property but the fundamental reality.
- The world of objects is seen as appearances within consciousness rather than independent realities. This concept has deep implications about the consciousness permeating all objects of our observation. This includes our body, mind and objects of this world. Cosciousness may be considered as ocean's water and objects of this world as waves manifesting on ocean surface. Essentially both ocean and waves are water. This close relationship of consciousness and the manifested world makes the interaction between the two possible. Through our thoughts in our mind, we can cause effects on our body. This is the basis for the power of thoughts on our body processes.

The Witness Consciousness

- The concept of Sakshi (witness) consciousness that observes but does not engage with experiences.

- The practice of cultivating witness awareness in meditation and daily life. By cultivating witness awareness we can remain unaffected by the ups and downs of our life. This state is ultimate goal of human life. However, use of thoughts to create positive outcomes in our body is a practical application of this profound law of nature.

Consciousness and Maya

- The role of consciousness in the creation and perception of the illusory world (Maya).
- How ignorance (Avidya) veils the true nature of consciousness as Brahman? As per Advaita Vedanta[4] the ignorance is the cause of our bondage and our inability to perceive the true nature of reality. Ignorance (Avidya) can be removed by following the stipulated spiritual path.

Yoga and the Science of Consciousness

- Patanjali's Yoga Sutras as a systematic approach to understanding and exploring consciousness.
- The goal of Yoga as the stilling of mental modifications to reveal pure consciousness.

Comparative Analysis: Scientific and Hindu Views on Consciousness

Despite their different methodologies and contexts, scientific and Hindu approaches to consciousness offer some intriguing parallels and contrasts:

The Primacy of Consciousness

- Some interpretations of quantum mechanics suggest a fundamental role for consciousness in reality.

---

[4] *https://www.britannica.com/topic/Advaita-school-of-Hindu-philosophy*

- Hindu philosophy, particularly Advaita Vedanta, posits consciousness as the ultimate reality.

The Observer Effect

- The role of the observer in quantum mechanics has parallels with the concept of witness consciousness in Hindu thought.

- Both perspectives challenge the notion of an objective reality independent of consciousness.

Unity of Consciousness

- Some scientific theories propose an integrated or unified nature of consciousness (e.g., Integrated Information Theory).

- Hindu philosophy often describes a fundamental unity of all consciousness in Brahman.

Altered States of Consciousness

- Scientific interest in meditation, psychedelics, and other altered states aligns with Hindu explorations of different levels of consciousness.

- Both approaches recognize the potential for expanded or transcendent states of awareness.

The Hard Problem of Consciousness[5]

- The scientific struggle with the hard problem of consciousness resonates with the Hindu recognition of consciousness as ultimately mysterious and self-revealing. The "hard problem of consciousness" asks how physical processes in the brain give rise to subjective, qualitative experiences (qualia). It contrasts with "easy problems" of explaining how the brain performs cognitive functions like behavior, information integration, and discrimination. Essentially, it's the question of why and how neural activity leads to a "something it is like" experience.

---

[5] *https://iep.utm.edu/hard-problem-of-conciousness/*

Consciousness and Reality

- Some scientific perspectives (e.g., Wheeler's participatory universe) suggest a role for consciousness in shaping reality.
- Hindu philosophy often describes the manifest world as a play of consciousness (Lila).

Creation as an Act of Consciousness

- Hindu cosmologies often describe creation as a manifestation or dream of cosmic consciousness.
- Parallels with scientific notions of reality as information or computation.

The Evolution of Consciousness

- Scientific perspectives on the emergence and evolution of consciousness in the cosmos.
- Hindu views on the unfoldment of consciousness through different forms and levels of manifestation.

Philosophical Implications

The study of consciousness raises profound philosophical questions that bridge scientific and spiritual inquiries:

The Nature of Self

- How does our understanding of consciousness affect our concept of self?
- The Buddhist doctrine of Anatta (no-self) and its relevance to both scientific and Hindu views.

Free Will and Determinism

- How does consciousness relate to questions of free will?
- Reconciling apparent free will with both physical laws and the concept of a unified consciousness.

The Mind-Body Problem

- Various approaches to understanding the relationship between consciousness and physical reality.

- Parallels between scientific theories of mind-body relationship and Hindu concepts of subtle bodies.

Ethics and Consciousness

- How might our understanding of consciousness inform our ethical frameworks?
- The concept of expanded circles of compassion based on the unity of consciousness.

The Limits of Knowledge

- Can consciousness fully understand itself?
- The role of direct experience versus conceptual knowledge in understanding consciousness.

Practical Applications and Implications

How do these perspectives on consciousness translate into practical approaches and implications?

Meditation and Consciousness Exploration

- Scientific studies on the effects of meditation on the brain and consciousness.
- Hindu practices for exploring and expanding consciousness.

Consciousness in Healthcare

- The role of consciousness in healing and wellbeing.
- Integrating consciousness-based approaches with modern medicine. Our book is attempting to explore this possibility.
- Ethical considerations in the development of AI and potential artificial consciousness.

Conclusion: Consciousness as a Bridge

As we've explored in this chapter, consciousness serves as a crucial bridge between scientific and spiritual approaches to understanding the cosmos. Both perspectives recognize consciousness as a fundamental mystery, central to our experience of reality and potentially to the nature of reality itself.

The scientific study of consciousness, while still in its early stages, is revealing the profound complexity of awareness and its intimate relationship with the physical world. From the role of the observer in quantum mechanics to the global integration of information in the brain, science is uncovering layers of subtlety in how consciousness operates and relates to the world.

Hindu philosophy, with its millennia-long exploration of consciousness, offers profound insights into the nature of awareness, its potential states and dimensions, and its relationship to ultimate reality. The concept of consciousness as fundamental, rather than emergent, challenges materialist assumptions and opens up new ways of conceiving the cosmos.

The convergence of scientific and contemplative approaches to consciousness holds immense potential for deepening our understanding of ourselves and the universe.

2. The Science of Self-Healing

Introduction

In the quiet space between stimulus and response lies a power that many of us have yet to fully harness. This power—the ability of the mind to influence the body at the cellular level—represents one of the most fascinating frontiers in modern science. Yet paradoxically, it also reflects ancient wisdom traditions that have understood the mind-body connection for millennia in Hindu and other major religions.

The Taittiriya Upanishad from ancient Hindu thoughts describes in 'The Panch Kosha Vivek' (discrimination of the five sheaths) that the human being is composed of five nested layers or sheaths (koshas) that veil the true Self (Atman). Figure 1 below describes the concept pictorially[6].

1. **Annamaya Kosha (Food Sheath)** The outermost layer consisting of the physical body made from and sustained by food. It's the gross matter that experiences birth, growth, decay, and death. This sheath is temporary and subject to constant change.

2. **Pranamaya Kosha (Vital Air Sheath)** The energy body comprising the five vital airs (pranas) and the five organs of action. This sheath animates the physical body and includes breathing, circulation, and other vital functions. It's more subtle than the food sheath but still not the true Self.

---

[6] *https://ijip.in/wp-content/uploads/2020/06/18.01.105.20180602.pdf*

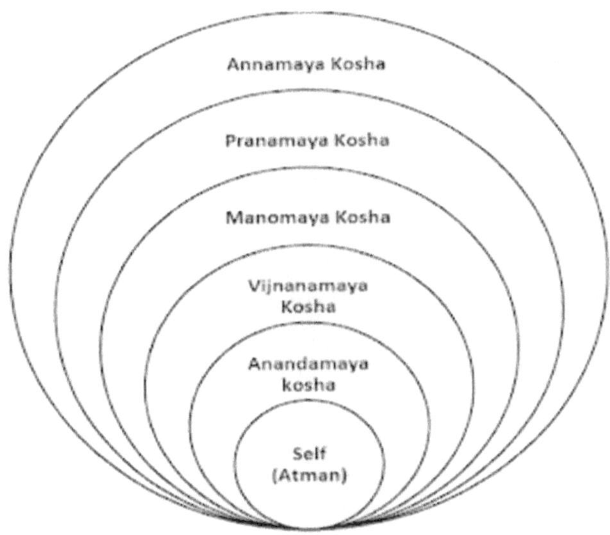

Fig 1: The pictorial view of five Sheaths that constitute our personality

3. **Manomaya Kosha (Mental Sheath)** The mind-body consisting of thoughts, emotions, and the five sense organs. This includes the thinking mind (manas) and encompasses desires, fears, anger, and other mental modifications. It's the seat of individual personality and ego-identification.

4. **Vijnanamaya Kosha (Intellectual Sheath)** The wisdom body containing the discriminating intellect (buddhi), ego (ahamkara), and deeper understanding. This is where discernment between real and unreal occurs, and where spiritual knowledge is processed. It's subtler than the mental sheath.

5. **Anandamaya Kosha (Bliss Sheath)** The innermost sheath of pure bliss and joy, closest to the Atman. It is experienced in meditation, and moments of profound peace. Though subtler than all others, it's still a covering over the true Self.

Most of us are normally beset by the physical and mental ailments that seem to be affecting our first three outer layers i.e. Annamaya, Pranamaya and Manomaya koshas. Meditation process puts us in contact with our innermost layer called Anandmaya. Each inner layer is subtler than the outer. Thus our body functions are controlled by the vital air and mental layers and mental layer is controlled by the intellectual layer. The meditative process puts us in a vantage position with respect to lower layers and subtle suggestions from the bliss layer may have desired effects in our body-mind complex.

This book plans to explore the intersection of two revolutionary scientific perspectives: the placebo effect as a demonstration of the mind's healing capacity, and telomere biology as a measurable indicator of cellular aging and renewal. By weaving these concepts together through the practice of meditation, we plan to unlock a pathway to not just manage stress or find momentary peace, but potentially influence the very mechanisms that determine how our cells age and regenerate.

The Placebo Effect: Mind Over Matter
The word "placebo" often conjures images of sugar pills and control groups—scientific footnotes rather than healing forces. Yet this perspective misses the profound implications of what placebo responses actually represent: the body's innate capacity for self-repair when the mind believes healing is occurring.

Dr. Joe Dispenza, in his groundbreaking work 'You Are the Placebo', reframes our understanding of this phenomenon. "The placebo effect," he writes, "is not about the sugar pill or the saline solution or the sham surgery. Those are just the vehicles used to elicit a thought. The placebo effect is an example of how powerful your thoughts can be."

Consider the landmark study by Dr. Bruce Moseley published in the New England Journal of Medicine in 2002[7]. Patients with severe, debilitating knee pain were divided into three groups. One received standard arthroscopic surgery to clear damaged cartilage, another received lavage surgery (where the knee joint is rinsed with saline), and the third received a sham surgery—patients were sedated, received incisions, and surgeons talked and moved as if performing the procedure, but no actual surgical intervention occurred.

The results were stunning: all three groups reported similar levels of pain reduction and improved mobility. Those who received sham surgery—who simply believed they had been treated—experienced the same benefits as those who underwent actual surgical interventions.

The Biochemistry of Belief

When you wholeheartedly accept that healing is occurring, your brain doesn't distinguish between an actual treatment and the belief in that treatment. It responds by producing the same chemical messengers—neurotransmitters, hormones, and peptides—that would be triggered by "real" interventions.

These biochemical messengers circulate throughout your body, binding to receptors on cell membranes and triggering cascades

---

7 https://www.nejm.org/doi/full/10.1056/NEJMoa013259

of cellular activity. In essence, your expectation of healing becomes a molecular instruction set for your cells.

Research has shown that placebo responses can:

- Stimulate the release of endorphins, the body's natural painkillers
- Reduce inflammatory responses by modulating immune function
- Activate reward pathways in the brain that promote healing and resilience
- Trigger the parasympathetic nervous system (rest and digest mode)
- Influence gene expression related to stress response, inflammation, and cellular repair

Telomeres: The Timekeepers of Cellular Age

While the placebo effect demonstrates the mind's influence over bodily processes, telomere biology gives us a measurable way to track how well our cells are aging. Discovered by Elizabeth Blackburn (who later won the Nobel Prize for this work), telomeres are the protective caps at the ends of our chromosomes, similar to the plastic tips on shoelaces.

Each time a cell divides, these telomeres become slightly shorter. When they reach a critical length, the cell either becomes senescent (enters a zombie-like state where it no longer functions properly but refuses to die) or undergoes apoptosis (programmed cell death). This progressive shortening of telomeres is one of the primary mechanisms of aging.

What makes telomeres particularly fascinating is that their rate of shortening isn't fixed.

Various factors can accelerate or slow telomere attrition:

1. **Chronic stress**: Psychological stress triggers fight-or-flight responses that, when chronic, lead to accelerated telomere shortening.

2. **Inflammation**: Persistent inflammatory states, often linked to stress, poor diet, and environmental factors, can speed telomere erosion.

3. **Oxidative damage**: Free radicals damage telomeric DNA more readily than other parts of chromosomes.

4. **Lifestyle factors**: Diet, exercise, sleep quality, and social connection all influence telomere maintenance.

5. **Mental states**: Remarkably, negative thought patterns, rumination, and pessimism correlate with shorter telomeres.

As Dr. Elizabeth Blackburn and Dr. Elissa Epel write in The Telomere Effect: "The foods you eat, your response to emotional challenges, the amount of exercise you get, whether you were exposed to childhood stress, and even the level of trust and safety in your neighbourhood—all of these factors and more appear to influence your telomeres and can prevent premature aging at the cellular level."

The Telomerase Solution

If telomere shortening represents the ticking clock of cellular aging, might there be a way to slow or even reverse this process? This is where telomerase enters the picture.

Telomerase is an enzyme that can add DNA sequences back to shortened telomeres, essentially rewinding the cellular aging clock. While most of our cells produce little telomerase after early development (which is actually protective against cancer), research suggests that we may be able to influence telomerase activity through lifestyle and psychological factors.

This brings us to the remarkable intersection of the placebo effect and telomere biology—and the practice that might help us leverage both: **meditation**.

A groundbreaking study by Dr. Dean Ornish and colleagues published in The Lancet Oncology demonstrated that a comprehensive lifestyle intervention including meditation, dietary changes, moderate exercise, and social support led to a 30% increase in telomerase activity after just three months[8].

The Meditation Bridge

Meditation serves as the perfect bridge between the placebo effect and telomere biology for several reasons:

1. **Mind-Body Integration**: Meditation directly addresses the mind's ability to influence bodily processes—the very mechanism behind the placebo effect.

2. **Stress Reduction**: By activating the parasympathetic nervous system, meditation counteracts the stress responses that accelerate telomere shortening.

3. **Epigenetic Influence**: Research suggests that meditative practices may influence gene expression, potentially including genes that regulate telomerase activity.

4. **Present-Moment Awareness**: By reducing rumination and worry about the past and future, meditation may reduce the psychological states associated with telomere attrition.

---

[8] *Ornish D, Lin J, Daubenmier J, Weidner G, Epel E, Kemp C, Magbanua MJ, Marlin R, Yglecias L, Carroll PR, Blackburn EH. "Increased telomerase activity and comprehensive lifestyle changes: a pilot study". Lancet Oncol. 2008 Nov;9(11):1048-57. doi: 10.1016/S1470-2045(08)70234-1. Epub 2008 Sep 15. Erratum in: Lancet Oncol. 2008 Dec;9(12):1124. PMID: 18799354.*

5. **Neuroplastic Changes**: Regular meditation practice creates structural and functional changes in brain regions involved in self-regulation, emotional processing, and stress response.

The illustrative research findings[9], suggest that meditation may be more than just a relaxation technique—it could be a biological intervention that influences the very mechanisms of cellular aging[10].

The Mind as Medicine: A New Paradigm

When we integrate these scientific perspectives, a new paradigm emerges: the mind as medicine. This isn't merely positive thinking or wishful visualization. Rather, it's the recognition that consciousness itself may be a biological force—one that can influence gene expression, modulate immune function, regulate stress responses, and potentially even affect how our cells age. This perspective doesn't diminish the value of conventional medical treatments. Instead, it suggests that our internal mental environment creates a biological context that can either amplify or diminish the effectiveness of any intervention, whether pharmaceutical, surgical, or lifestyle-based.

---

[9] *Jacobs TL, Epel ES, Lin J, Blackburn EH, Wolkowitz OM, Bridwell DA, Zanesco AP, Aichele SR, Sahdra BK, MacLean KA, King BG, Shaver PR, Rosenberg EL, Ferrer E, Wallace BA, Saron CD. "Intensive meditation training, immune cell telomerase activity, and psychological mediators". Psychoneuroendocrinology. 2011 Jun;36(5):664-81. doi: 10.1016/j.psyneuen.2010.09.010. Epub 2010 Oct 29. PMID: 21035949.*

[10] *Elizabeth A. Hoge, Maxine M. Chen, Esther Orr, Christina A. Metcalf, Laura E. Fischer, Mark H. Pollack, Immaculata DeVivo, Naomi M. Simon, "Loving-Kindness Meditation practice associated with longer telomeres in women", Brain, Behavior, and Immunity, Volume 32,2013,Pages 159-163,ISSN 0889-1591,https://doi.org/10.1016/j.bbi.2013.04.005.(https://www.sciencedirect.com/science/article/pii/S0889159113001736)*

Dr. Dispenza puts it this way: "The latest research supports the notion that we have a natural ability to change the brain and body by thought alone... mental rehearsal can change brain circuitry, and thus we can change our brains just by thinking differently."

A Personal Practice: Beginning our Journey
We stand at the threshold of a new understanding of human potential—one that honours both ancient wisdom and cutting-edge science. Throughout this book, we'll explore practical ways to apply these insights through increasingly refined meditation practices designed to influence telomere maintenance, activate self-healing responses, and create an optimal internal environment for cellular health.
The human consciousness as conceptualised in 'Panch Kosh Vivek' (refer Figure 1 above) manifests through the highest layer i.e. Blissful layer down to all lower layers culminating in body layer and is considered to have deep effect on all aspects of human personality.

The science of self-healing is not about rejecting conventional medicine or embracing magical thinking. It's about recognizing and leveraging the powerful biological mechanisms that connect mind and body—mechanisms that have always been there, waiting for us to use them consciously.

Understanding these concepts intellectually is one thing; experiencing their reality in our own life is another. Practice of meditation towards the set objectives is crucial to success.

Conclusion: The Journey Ahead

We stand at the threshold of a new understanding of human potential—one that honors both ancient wisdom and cutting-edge science. Throughout this book, we'll explore practical ways to apply these insights through increasingly refined meditation practices designed to influence telomere maintenance, activate self-healing responses, and create an optimal internal environment for cellular health.

The journey ahead isn't about quick fixes or miracle cures. It's about developing a consistent practice that aligns your consciousness with your biology, creating the conditions for optimal cellular renewal. As we'll discover in subsequent chapters, this alignment can influence everything from stress responses to sleep quality, from inflammatory processes to genetic expression.

The science of self-healing isn't about rejecting conventional medicine or embracing magical thinking. It's about recognizing and leveraging the powerful biological mechanisms that connect mind and body—mechanisms that have always been there, waiting for us to use them consciously.

In the next chapter, we'll dive deeper into telomere biology and explore the specific cellular pathways influenced by meditation practice. For now, I encourage you to practice the simple awareness meditation daily, beginning the process of conscious dialogue with your cells.

As we conclude this chapter, I invite you to try a simple meditation practice that will begin to build the bridge between these scientific insights and your lived experience.

Basic Awareness Meditation (5-10 minutes)

1. Find a comfortable seated position where your spine can be straight but relaxed. Close your eyes or maintain a soft gaze.

2. Bring awareness to your breath, noticing the natural rhythm without trying to change it. Feel the sensation of air moving in and out of your body.

3. As you continue breathing naturally, imagine each breath bringing renewal to every cell in your body. Visualize your cells responding to this conscious attention—perhaps as tiny lights becoming brighter with each breath.

4. When your mind wanders (which is natural and expected), gently notice this without judgment and return your attention to your breath and the sensation of cellular renewal.

5. After 5-10 minutes, slowly bring your awareness back to the room, opening your eyes if they were closed.

This simple practice begins the process of directing conscious awareness to cellular processes—the foundation for the more advanced practices we'll explore in later chapters.

Reflection Questions

1. Have you ever experienced a placebo response or witnessed the mind's influence over physical symptoms? What were the circumstances?

2. What aspects of your current lifestyle might be influencing your telomere health, positively or negatively?

3. What barriers might prevent you from establishing a regular meditation practice, and how might you address them?

4. When you practiced the awareness meditation, what sensations or experiences did you notice?

5. How does the concept of "mind as medicine" challenge or complement your current understanding of health and healing?

3. Understanding Your Inner Biology

Introduction

When you look in the mirror, you see a singular being—your body, your face, your unique features. Yet this apparent unity masks an astonishing truth: you are composed of approximately 37 trillion cells, each a miniature living system with its own complex processes. These cells are constantly communicating, dividing, repairing, and responding to their environment. And at the heart of each cell lies your DNA—the blueprint of life itself.

In this chapter, we dive deeper into the invisible world within you, focusing on telomeres—the protective caps at the ends of your chromosomes that function as biological timekeepers. By understanding these molecular structures and how they respond to your thoughts, emotions, and behaviors, you gain insight into one of the most fundamental mechanisms of aging and renewal. This understanding forms the foundation for applying meditative practices to influence your cellular health. Figures below courtesy freepik.com show various illustrative cells in our body and anatomy of a cell.

Telomeres: The Protective Timekeepers

Imagine the shoelaces in your favorite pair of running shoes. At each end is a plastic or metal aglet that prevents the lace from fraying. Telomeres serve a similar purpose for your chromosomes—they are specialized structures composed of repetitive DNA sequences (TTAGGG in humans) that protect the ends of chromosomes from deterioration.

As Dr. Elizabeth Blackburn, who won the Nobel Prize for discovering telomerase, explains: "Telomeres are like the little

Cells of The Human Body

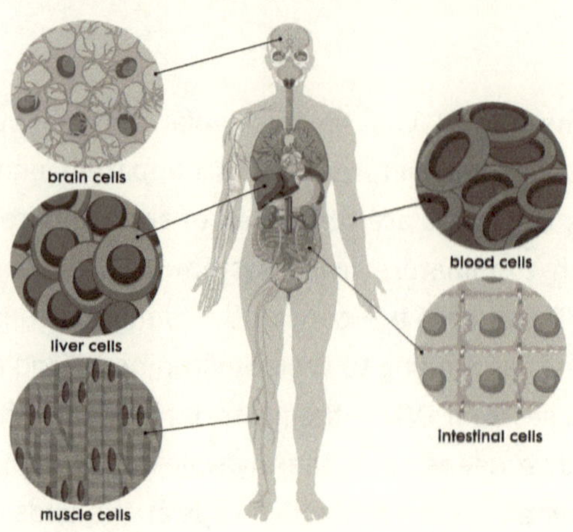

plastic tips on the ends of shoelaces. They keep chromosome ends from fraying and sticking to each other, which would destroy or scramble genetic information." Every time a cell divides—which happens millions of times daily throughout your body—the DNA must be replicated. Due to the mechanics of DNA replication, a small portion at the end of each chromosome cannot be copied. This is known as the "end replication problem." Telomeres serve as a buffer zone, sacrificing some of their length with each division to protect the crucial genetic information within the chromosome.

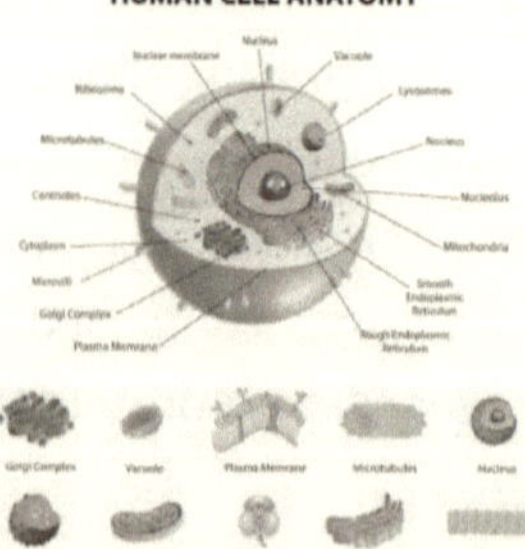

Over time, as telomeres progressively shorten, cells eventually reach a critical point called the "Hayflick limit," named after the scientist who first observed that normal human cells can only divide a certain number of times before stopping. At this point, cells typically do one of three things:

1. **Enter senescence**: The cell stops dividing but remains metabolically active, often secreting inflammatory compounds that damage neighboring cells.

2. **Undergo apoptosis**: The cell activates a programmed cell death pathway, essentially sacrificing itself for the greater good of the organism.

3. **Become dysfunctional**: In rare cases, cells with critically short telomeres may continue dividing by bypassing normal cellular checkpoints, potentially leading to genomic instability and cancer.

This telomere shortening process correlates strongly with biological aging. Studies have found that people with shorter telomeres tend to show more signs of aging and have higher risks for age-related diseases, including cardiovascular disease, diabetes, cancer, and neurodegenerative conditions.

Telomerase: The Renewal Enzyme

If telomere shortening represents a ticking clock counting down to cellular senescence, is there any way to slow or reverse this process? The answer lies in an extraordinary enzyme called telomerase.

Telomerase, also discovered by Dr. Blackburn along with Carol Greider and Jack Szostak, is an enzyme that can add DNA sequences back onto telomeres. It carries its own RNA template and uses it to synthesize new telomeric DNA, essentially rewinding the cellular aging clock.

In most adult human cells, telomerase activity is strictly regulated and generally kept low. This makes evolutionary sense— unlimited cell division could increase cancer risk. However, certain cells maintain active telomerase throughout life, including:

- **Stem cells**: Which need to divide repeatedly to replenish tissues
- **Immune cells**: Particularly when they need to proliferate rapidly to fight infection
- **Reproductive cells**: Which must maintain their telomere length to pass on to the next generation

The discovery that telomerase activity isn't fixed but can be modulated under certain conditions opened a fascinating possibility: What if we could influence telomerase activity through our lifestyle choices, psychological states, and practices like meditation?

Research has begun to suggest that this might indeed be possible. A pioneering study by Dr. Dean Ornish and colleagues found that a comprehensive lifestyle intervention—including meditation, dietary changes, exercise, and social support—was associated with a significant increase in telomerase activity after just three months.

Similarly, research from the laboratory of Dr. Elissa Epel and Dr. Elizabeth Blackburn found that chronic psychological stress was associated with lower telomerase activity and shorter telomeres. This suggests that stress reduction techniques, including meditation, might help maintain telomere length.

Stress Response Pathways: The Cellular Impact of Your Thoughts

To understand how meditation might influence telomere biology, we need to explore how stress affects your cells. When you experience stress—whether physical danger or psychological pressure—your body activates several interrelated pathways:

The HPA Axis: Your Body's Stress Response System

The hypothalamic-pituitary-adrenal (HPA) axis is your body's primary stress response system. When you perceive a threat, your hypothalamus releases corticotropin-releasing hormone (CRH), which triggers your pituitary gland to release adrenocorticotropic hormone (ACTH). This hormone then stimulates your adrenal glands to produce cortisol—your primary stress hormone.

Cortisol has numerous effects throughout your body, including:
- Increasing blood glucose to provide immediate energy
- Suppressing non-essential functions like digestion and reproduction
- Modulating immune system activity
- Affecting brain function, particularly in regions involved in emotional processing and memory

While this response is adaptive in the short term, chronic activation of the HPA axis can lead to dysregulation, with significant consequences for cellular health. Research has shown that chronically elevated cortisol levels correlate with accelerated telomere shortening.

Oxidative Stress: Free Radical Damage

Another critical pathway through which stress affects telomeres is oxidative stress. When your cells produce energy, they generate byproducts called reactive oxygen species (ROS) or free radicals. Under normal conditions, your body neutralizes these molecules through antioxidant defenses.

However, psychological stress increases free radical production while potentially depleting antioxidant reserves. These free radicals can damage cellular components, including DNA. Importantly, telomeric DNA is particularly vulnerable to oxidative damage—up to ten times more susceptible than non-telomeric DNA.

Inflammation: The Silent Cellular Fire

The third major pathway connecting stress to telomere health is inflammation. Psychological stress activates inflammatory signaling, increasing the production of pro-inflammatory cytokines—messenger molecules that coordinate immune responses.

Chronic inflammation creates a cellular environment that accelerates telomere shortening through multiple mechanisms:

- Direct damage to telomeric DNA
- Increased cell turnover, forcing more divisions
- Reduced telomerase activity
- Amplification of oxidative stress

Research has shown that inflammatory markers like interleukin-6 (IL-6) and C-reactive protein (CRP) correlate with shorter telomeres. Importantly, meditation has been shown to reduce these inflammatory markers, potentially protecting telomere integrity.

The Telomere Integration Model: How Your Life Affects Your Cells

Based on the complex interplay between psychological experience and cellular biology, researchers have developed what might be called the "Telomere Integration Model." This model helps us understand how various aspects of our lives—from stress and emotions to sleep and nutrition—ultimately influence our telomeres.

Psychological Factors

Perceived Stress: Your subjective experience of stress matters more than objective stressors. Studies show that people who perceive their lives as highly stressful tend to have shorter telomeres, regardless of actual life circumstances.

Rumination and Thought Patterns: Dwelling on negative experiences, catastrophizing, and pessimistic thinking styles are associated with shorter telomeres. This suggests that the quality of your thoughts—not just your external circumstances—impacts cellular aging.

Depression and Anxiety: Clinical studies have found that depression and anxiety disorders correlate with accelerated telomere shortening, possibly through chronic activation of stress response systems.

Behavioral Factors

Sleep Quality: Poor sleep—whether insufficient duration or disrupted quality—is linked to shorter telomeres. During deep sleep, your body activates many repair processes, including those that may help maintain telomere integrity.

Physical Activity: Regular moderate exercise is consistently associated with longer telomeres. Exercise likely protects telomeres through multiple mechanisms, including reduced inflammation, improved stress regulation, and enhanced antioxidant defenses.

Nutrition: Dietary patterns affect telomere health. Mediterranean-style diets rich in omega-3 fatty acids, antioxidants, and plant compounds are associated with better telomere maintenance, while processed foods high in refined sugars and unhealthy fats correlate with shorter telomeres.

Social Factors

Social Connection: Strong social bonds appear protective for telomeres. Studies show that people with better social support tend to have longer telomeres, while loneliness and social isolation correlate with telomere attrition.

Early Life Experiences: Childhood adversity can leave a lasting imprint on telomere biology. Research has found that traumatic childhood experiences are associated with shorter telomeres in adulthood, suggesting early programming of cellular aging trajectories.

Purpose and Meaning: Having a sense of purpose and meaning in life correlates with longer telomeres, possibly by buffering against stress and promoting healthier behaviors.

The Cellular Benefits of Meditation

Given our understanding of telomere biology and stress response pathways, meditation emerges as a powerful potential intervention for cellular health. Research has begun to elucidate specific mechanisms through which meditation may influence telomere maintenance:

Stress Reduction

At the most fundamental level, meditation reduces activation of stress response systems. Regular practice has been shown to:

- Lower baseline cortisol levels
- Reduce amygdala reactivity to stressors
- Improve recovery from stress exposures
- Decrease autonomic nervous system activation

These changes create a physiological environment more conducive to telomere maintenance and potentially higher telomerase activity.

Reducing Oxidative Stress

Multiple studies have found that various forms of meditation increase antioxidant activity while reducing markers of oxidative stress. By neutralizing free radicals more effectively, meditation may help protect telomeric DNA from oxidative damage.

Modulating Inflammation

Research consistently shows that meditation practices reduce inflammatory markers, including:

- Interleukin-6 (IL-6)
- C-reactive protein (CRP)

- Nuclear factor kappa B (NF-κB), a master regulator of inflammation

By dampening chronic inflammation, meditation may create a cellular milieu that supports rather than undermines telomere integrity.

Epigenetic Effects

Perhaps most fascinating are studies suggesting that meditation influences epigenetic patterns—changes in gene expression that don't alter the underlying DNA sequence. Research has found that experienced meditators show different methylation patterns in genes related to stress response, inflammation, and cellular aging.

This suggests that meditation may "turn up" genes that support cellular health while "turning down" genes that accelerate aging processes, potentially including those that regulate telomerase activity.

Key Meditation Studies on Telomere Biology

Several pioneering studies have directly examined the relationship between meditation practices and telomere biology:

The Shamatha Project

In this comprehensive study, participants attended a three-month intensive meditation retreat focusing on concentration practices. Compared to a control group, retreat participants showed significantly increased telomerase activity at the end of the retreat.

Mindfulness-Based Stress Reduction (MBSR) Research

Multiple studies of MBSR—an eight-week structured mindfulness program—have found associations with:

- Preserved telomere length compared to control groups

- Increased telomerase activity following the program

- Changes in gene expression related to telomere maintenance

Loving-Kindness Meditation Effects

A study examining loving-kindness meditation (focusing on generating feelings of compassion) found that participants had longer telomeres compared to controls, with the difference particularly pronounced in women.

These findings, while preliminary, suggest that various forms of meditation may indeed influence the biology of cellular aging through telomere maintenance.

Your Inner Ecosystem: Beyond Telomeres

While telomeres provide a valuable lens for understanding cellular aging, they're part of a broader inner ecosystem that meditation can influence. Other important cellular mechanisms affected by meditation include:

Mitochondrial Function

Mitochondria—the cellular "power plants" that generate energy—are crucial for healthy aging. Chronic stress impairs mitochondrial function, while meditation appears to support mitochondrial biogenesis (the creation of new mitochondria) and efficiency.

Cellular Senescence Factors

Beyond telomere shortening, cells can enter senescence through other pathways. Meditation may reduce these alternate senescence triggers, including genotoxic stress (DNA damage) and mitochondrial dysfunction.

Neural Stem Cell Activity

In the brain, neural stem cells help maintain cognitive function with age. Stress reduces neural stem cell proliferation, while preliminary research suggests meditation may support their activity.

Putting Knowledge Into Practice: Your Cellular Awareness Meditation

Understanding telomere biology and stress response pathways provides a scientific foundation for meditation practice. With this knowledge, you can approach meditation not just as a relaxation technique, but as a biological intervention—a way of communicating with your 37 trillion cells.

Here is a practice designed specifically to bring awareness to your cellular biology:

Cellular Renewal Meditation (15-20 minutes)

1. Find a comfortable seated position where your spine can be straight but relaxed. Close your eyes or maintain a soft gaze.

2. Begin by bringing awareness to your breath, allowing it to deepen naturally. With each inhale, imagine bringing fresh oxygen and nutrients to your cells. With each exhale, visualize your cells releasing waste products and cellular debris.

3. Bring your attention to your heart space. Feel your heartbeat—the rhythm that has been sustaining your life since before your birth. Recognize that this steady beat delivers blood to every one of your trillions of cells.

4. Now visualize your chromosomes within your cells—the thread-like structures containing your DNA. At the ends of each chromosome are your telomeres—the protective caps that preserve your genetic information.

5. Imagine these telomeres glowing with a soft, healing light. As you continue breathing deeply, visualize this light growing stronger with each breath, representing the activation of telomerase and cellular repair mechanisms.

6. Bring awareness to any areas of tension or stress in your body. Notice how stress affects your physical sensations. As you breathe into these areas, imagine your cells releasing stress hormones and inflammatory compounds.

7. Now visualize your entire cellular network shifting from a state of stress response to a state of renewal. See your telomeres stabilizing, protected by the physiological changes triggered by your meditation.

8. Spend several minutes resting in this awareness of cellular renewal. Trust in your body's innate wisdom and capacity for self-repair.

9. Before completing the practice, set an intention to carry this cellular awareness with you throughout your day—remembering that each thought, emotion, and choice influences your telomeres and cellular health.

10. Slowly bring your awareness back to the room, opening your eyes if they were closed.

This meditation combines visualization with actual physiological changes that occur during meditative states. By practicing regularly, you're not merely imagining cellular renewal—you're creating the biological conditions that support it.

Conclusion: The Conscious Cell

Throughout this chapter, we've explored the intimate connection between your conscious experience and your cellular biology. Telomeres—those tiny caps at the ends of your chromosomes—serve as a biological bridge between mind and body, responding to your thoughts, emotions, behaviors, and practices.

The research on meditation and telomere biology suggests something profound: your consciousness may be a biological force—capable of influencing genetic expression, cellular repair mechanisms, and the very trajectory of aging itself.

This doesn't mean meditation is a miracle cure or that we can completely halt aging through thought alone. Rather, it suggests that by developing awareness and skillfully working with your mind, you can create an internal environment more conducive to cellular health and resilience.

In the next chapter, we'll explore different meditation traditions and their approaches, examining how various techniques affect different aspects of brain function and physiology. This understanding will help you develop a personalized practice that addresses your unique biological needs.

For now, I encourage you to practice the Cellular Renewal Meditation daily, beginning a conscious dialogue with the trillions of cells that comprise your physical being. Remember that each session is an opportunity to shift your physiology from stress response to renewal—with potential benefits extending all the way to the tips of your chromosomes.

Reflection Questions

1. Were you surprised by any of the connections between psychological experience and cellular biology? Which findings resonated most strongly with you?

2. Reflecting on your life, can you identify periods when stress might have accelerated your cellular aging? What about periods of renewal when you might have supported telomere maintenance?

3. How does the knowledge that your thoughts and emotions Influence your cells at a molecular level change how you view your meditation practice?

4. When practicing the Cellular Renewal Meditation, what sensations or insights arose? Did you notice any difference in your stress levels before and after?

5. Beyond meditation, what other aspects of your lifestyle might you adjust to better support telomere health and cellular renewal?

4. The Power of Meditation

Introduction

In the previous chapters, we explored how thoughts and emotions influence cellular health through telomere biology and stress response pathways. Now we turn our attention to the practice that allows us to consciously engage with these processes: **meditation**. While meditation is often presented as a singular technique, it actually encompasses a rich variety of approaches, each with its own focus, methodology, and effects on brain and body.

Understanding these different traditions and their neurological impacts allows you to choose practices that best serve your needs and goals. Whether you seek stress reduction, emotional balance, cognitive enhancement, or cellular renewal, specific meditation techniques can help create the internal conditions you desire. It may be of interest to readers that meditation is inevitable step towards our spiritual journey too. It puts us in contact with our true self. Since the focus of this book is on our body and mind apparatus and use of our conscious thoughts/suggestions to achieve positive impact at the plane of our body and mind, we shall not continue to explore use of meditation in achieving our spiritual goals. However, any progress in this powerful technique towards our body and mind would help us maintain equanimity in our worldly life while facing the turbulences that are part of this world.

The Neuroscience Of Meditation: Overview

Before exploring specific traditions, let's understand what happens in the brain during meditation. Modern neuroscience has revealed that meditation creates distinct patterns of brain activity associated with:

Structural Changes

- Increased gray matter density in regions associated with attention, emotional regulation, and self-awareness
- Enhanced connectivity between brain regions involved in self-referential processing and emotional regulation
- Thickening of the cortex in areas related to attention and sensory processing

Functional Changes

- Reduced activity in the default mode network (DMN), associated with mind-wandering and self-referential thinking
- Increased activation in areas associated with attention and emotional regulation
- Enhanced communication between different brain networks
- Altered patterns of brain wave activity, particularly increased alpha and theta waves

Biochemical Changes

- Reduced levels of stress hormones like cortisol
- Increased production of neurotransmitters associated with well-being, including serotonin and GABA
- Changes in gene expression related to inflammation and stress response
- Increased telomerase activity in certain meditation practices

Core Meditation Traditions and Their Effects

Let's explore major meditation traditions and their specific impacts on brain and body:

1. **Focused Attention Meditation (Shamatha)**

Description: This fundamental practice involves maintaining attention on a single object—often the breath, a visual point, or a mantra. When attention wanders, it's gently brought back to the chosen focus.

Neural Effects:

- Strengthens anterior cingulate cortex, crucial for attention and self-regulation

- Enhances activity in the prefrontal cortex, supporting executive function

- Reduces default mode network activity, decreasing mind-wandering

- Increases gamma wave synchronization, associated with heightened awareness

Practice Example: Basic Breath Awarenes

1. Sit comfortably with your spine straight

2. Direct attention to the sensation of breathing at your nostrils or abdomen

3. When mind wanders, gently return attention to breath

4. Start with 5-10 minutes, gradually increasing duration

5. Note: This foundational practice develops concentration necessary for other techniques

2. Open Monitoring Meditation (Vipassana)

Description: This practice involves non-judgmental awareness of whatever arises in experience—thoughts, emotions, sensations—without becoming attached or reactive.

Neural Effects:

- Activates insula and anterior cingulate cortex, improving interoception and emotional awareness

- Reduces amygdala reactivity to emotional stimuli

- Enhances connectivity between prefrontal and limbic regions

- Increases theta wave activity, associated with deep relaxation and emotional processing

Practice Example: Body Scanning

1. Lie down or sit comfortably

2. Systematically move attention through body parts

3. Notice sensations without trying to change them

4. Maintain equanimous awareness of pleasant/unpleasant experiences

5. Practice for 20-30 minutes

3. **Loving-Kindness Meditation (Metta)**

Description: Focuses on cultivating feelings of compassion and goodwill toward self and others, starting with loved ones and gradually expanding to all beings.

Neural Effects:

- Activates regions associated with empathy and emotional processing

- Increases activity in left prefrontal cortex, associated with positive emotions

- Enhances vagal tone[11], improving autonomic nervous system regulation. Vagal tone refers to the level of activity in the vagus nerve, a major part of the parasympathetic nervous system. It's essentially a measure of the parasympathetic nervous system's influence on the heart and other bodily functions, and it's often used as a way to assess stress and stress vulnerability. High vagal tone is generally associated with greater adaptability and resilience, while low vagal tone can be linked to increased stress sensitivity and difficulties in regulating emotions and attention.

- Shows particular benefits for telomere maintenance in long-term practitioners

Practice Example: Expanding Circle of Compassion

---

[11] *https://www.massgeneral.org/news/article/vagus-nerve#*

1. Begin with self-directed well-wishes
2. Extend to loved ones
3. Include neutral persons
4. Embrace difficult relationships
5. Expand to all beings
6. Practice for 15-20 minutes

4. Transcendental Meditation (TM)

Description: Uses silent repetition of a personalized mantra to transcend ordinary thinking and access deeper states of consciousness.

Neural Effects:

- Increases alpha wave coherence across brain regions
- Reduces stress hormone production
- Enhances default mode network integration
- Shows significant effects on cellular aging markers

Note: TM requires instruction from certified teachers and uses personalized mantras.

5. Mindfulness-Based Stress Reduction (MBSR)

Description: An eight-week structured program combining mindfulness meditation, body awareness, and yoga.

Neural Effects:

- Reduces gray matter density in amygdala, associated with stress and anxiety
- Increases hippocampal volume, supporting memory and emotional regulation
- Shows beneficial effects on inflammatory markers and telomerase activity
- Improves immune system functioning

Core Components:

- Formal meditation practice
- Body scan exercises
- Gentle yoga

- Daily life mindfulness
- Group discussion and support

6. **Contemplative Inquiry**

Description: Uses directed questioning and meditation to investigate the nature of consciousness and experience.

Neural Effects:

- Activates regions associated with self-referential processing
- Enhances metacognitive awareness
- Shows unique patterns of default mode network modulation
- May support neuroplastic changes in self-processing networks

Practice Example: Self-Inquiry Meditation

1. Begin with focused attention to stabilize mind
2. Ask "Who am I?" or "What is aware of this experience?"
3. Rest in the space that opens with questioning
4. Notice what remains when thoughts subside
5. Practice for 20-30 minute

Advanced Meditation States and Their Effects

Long-term practitioners often report accessing distinct states of consciousness with unique neurological signatures:

1. **Flow States**

- Characterized by absorbed attention and effortless action
- Shows reduced activity in self-referential processing areas
- Increases theta wave activity
- Associated with peak performance and creativity

2. **Witness Consciousness**

- Maintained awareness during sleep states
- Unique EEG signatures combining delta and gamma waves
- Enhanced functional connectivity between normally distinct networks
- Reported improvements in sleep quality and daytime alertness

3. **Non-Dual Awareness**

- Dissolution of subject-object distinction
- Reduced activity in brain regions involved in self-other processing
- Increased global coherence across brain networks
- Associated with reports of unity consciousness

Establishing Your Practice: Guidelines for Success

To develop an effective meditation practice that supports cellular health and overall well-being:

1. **Start Gradually**
- Begin with 5-10 minutes daily
- Focus on consistency over duration
- Build up time slowly as concentration improves
- Expect and accept fluctuations in practice quality

2. **Create Supportive Conditions**
- Designate a quiet space for practice
- Practice at the same time daily
- Use comfortable but alert posture
- Consider joining a meditation group or class

3. **Address Common Challenges**
- Mind wandering is normal—return attention gently
- Physical discomfort—adjust posture mindfully
- Sleepiness—practice with eyes open or at different times
- Resistance—start with shorter sessions
- Expectations—focus on process over results

4. **Track Your Progress**
- Keep a meditation journal
- Note duration and type of practice
- Record insights and challenges
- Observe changes in daily life
- Consider using meditation apps for guidance

Integration Practice: The Three-Stage Meditation

This comprehensive practice combines elements from different traditions to support both cellular health and consciousness development:

Stage 1: Foundation (5-10 minutes)

1. Establish stable posture

2. Focus attention on breath

3. Develop concentration and presence

4. Allow body and mind to settle

Stage 2: Cellular Awareness (10-15 minutes)

1. Scan body systematically

2. Notice cellular activity and energy

3. Visualize telomere maintenance

4. Direct healing intention to areas of tension

Stage 3: Open Awareness (10-15 minutes)

1. Release all focus points

2. Rest in natural awareness

3. Allow experience to unfold freely

4. Notice the space of consciousness itself

Scientific Validation: Research Highlights

While "Cellular Renewal Meditation" isn't a specific, established term in scientific research, the underlying concepts of meditation and its potential impact on cellular health are supported by evidence[12]. Studies suggest that meditation, particularly mindfulness-based practices, can influence telomere length, telomerase activity, and overall cellular health. These effects are

---

[12] *I. Gusti Ngurah Putra Eka Santosa, I. Made Jawi, I. Made Bakta, I. Wayan Putu Sutirta Yasa, I. Made Ady Wirawan, Lesmana, C. B. J., Kandarini, Y., Susy Purnamawati, & Ida Bagus Yorky Brahmantya. (2024). The effect of meditation on telomerase and stem cell. International Journal of Research in Medical Sciences, 12(9), 3491–3499. https://doi.org/10.18203/2320-6012.ijrms20242638*

linked to stress reduction, improved immune function, and a reduction in oxidative stress[13].

Recent studies have demonstrated meditation's effects across multiple domains[14]:

Cognitive Function

- Improved attention and working memory
- Enhanced emotional regulation
- Better stress management
- Increased cognitive flexibility

Physical Health

- Reduced inflammation markers
- Improved immune function
- Better cardiovascular health
- Enhanced telomerase activity

Psychological Well-being

- Reduced anxiety and depression
- Increased life satisfaction
- Better emotional awareness
- Improved relationships

Cellular Health

- Preserved telomere length
- Reduced oxidative stress
- Improved mitochondrial function
- Enhanced cellular repair mechanisms

Building a Sustainable Practice

---

[13] *Dasanayaka, N.N., Sirisena, N.D. & Samaranayake, N. The effects of meditation on length of telomeres in healthy individuals: a systematic review. Syst Rev 10, 151 (2021). https://doi.org/10.1186/s13643-021-01699-1*

[14] *Epel E, Daubenmier J, Moskowitz JT, Folkman S, Blackburn E. Can meditation slow rate of cellular aging? Cognitive stress, mindfulness, and telomeres. Ann N Y Acad Sci. 2009 Aug;1172:34-53. doi: 10.1111/j.1749-6632.2009.04414.x. PMID: 19735238; PMCID: PMC3057175.*

To maintain a long-term meditation practice that supports cellular health:

1. Create a Practice Schedule

- Set realistic daily goals
- Plan for both formal and informal practice
- Include variety to maintain engagement
- Allow flexibility while maintaining consistency

2. Develop Supporting Habits

- Regular sleep schedule
- Healthy diet
- Regular exercise
- Stress management strategies

3. Join a Community

- Find local meditation groups
- Attend retreats when possible
- Share experiences with others
- Seek guidance when needed

4. Maintain Motivation

- Review scientific research
- Remember health benefits
- Connect with long-term practitioners
- Celebrate small improvements

Conclusion: The Path Forward

Understanding different meditation traditions and their effects allows you to choose practices that best support your goals for cellular health and consciousness development. Remember that meditation is both an art and a science—while we can measure its effects on brain and body, the subjective experience of practice remains deeply personal.

As you move forward, maintain both discipline and gentleness in your approach. Let the scientific understanding of meditation's benefits support your practice while remaining open to the direct experience of each moment.

In the next chapter, we'll explore how to break free from past conditioning that may accelerate cellular aging, using meditation to create new neural and emotional patterns that support health and longevity.

Reflection Questions

1. Which meditation tradition resonates most strongly with you? Why?

2. What challenges have you encountered in your meditation practice? How might you address them?

3. How does understanding the neuroscience of meditation influence your approach to practice?

4. What changes have you noticed since beginning meditation practice?

5. How might you integrate different meditation techniques to support your specific health and consciousness goals?

PART II

THE MIND AS MEDICINE

5.Breaking the Addiction to the Past

Introduction

Every thought you think, every emotion you feel, creates a biochemical response in your body. When thoughts and emotions become habitual, they create persistent biological states that can either support or undermine cellular health. As Dr. Joe Dispenza observes in "You Are the Placebo," many of us are "addicted" to past emotional states—unconsciously recreating the same biological conditions day after day, potentially accelerating cellular aging through chronic stress responses and inflammatory patterns.

This chapter explores how past conditioning influences your biology at the cellular level and provides specific meditation practices to break free from limiting patterns. By understanding and transforming these emotional-biochemical habits, you can create an internal environment more conducive to telomere maintenance and cellular renewal.

The Biology of Emotional Addiction
The Biochemical Signature of Emotions
Every emotional state[15] has a distinct biochemical signature involving:
- Neurotransmitters
- Hormones
- Neuropeptides
- Inflammatory markers

---

[15] Oatley, K., Keltner, D., & Jenkins, J. M. (2006). Understanding emotions (2nd ed.). Blackwell Publishing

- Gene expression patterns

When emotions become habitual, these biochemical patterns become your biological "default setting." Research has shown that:

1. **Chronic Stress Patterns**
   - Elevated cortisol levels
   - Increased inflammatory cytokines
   - Reduced telomerase activity
   - Accelerated telomere shortening

2. **Negative Emotional States**
   - Higher oxidative stress
   - Compromised immune function
   - Altered gene expression
   - Reduced cellular repair capacity

3. **Positive Emotional States**
   - Enhanced immune function
   - Increased DHEA (anti-aging hormone)
   - Improved cellular repair
   - Better telomere maintenance

Breaking the Cycle: The Neuroscience of Change

Neural Plasticity and Emotional Patterns

Your brain is constantly rewiring itself based on experience. When you repeatedly activate certain emotional circuits, you strengthen those neural pathways. However, the same plasticity that creates emotional habits can be used to break them.

Key aspects of neural remodeling:

1. **Hebbian Learning**
   - Neurons that fire together, wire together
   - Emotional patterns become self-reinforcing
   - New experiences can create new circuits

2. **Synaptic Pruning**
   - Unused circuits weaken over time

- Meditation can help "unwire" old patterns
- Active replacement creates lasting change

3. **State-Dependent Gene Expression**
   - Emotional states influence genetic activity
   - Chronic states create persistent patterns
   - Changing states can alter gene expression

The Meditation Protocol for Breaking Past Conditioning

Phase 1: Recognition and Awareness (15-20 minutes)

Practice Instructions:

1. Find a comfortable seated position
2. Close your eyes and focus on your breath
3. Scan your body for tension patterns
4. Notice recurring emotional states
5. Identify associated thoughts and memories
6. Observe without trying to change anything

Key Points:

- Build awareness of habitual patterns
- Notice physical manifestations of emotions
- Recognize recurring thought loops
- Stay present with discomfort

Phase 2: Release and Rewiring (20-30 minutes)

Practice Instructions:

1. Return to your emotional awareness
2. Locate emotions in your body
3. Practice the following sequence:

   a) **Acknowledge**
   - Name the emotion
   - Accept its presence
   - Release self-judgment

b) **Release**

- Breathe into the emotion

- Imagine tension dissolving

- Let go of the story

c) **Replace**

- Generate positive emotion

- Amplify the new state

- Anchor it in your body

4. Repeat with different emotional patterns

Phase 3: Cellular Renovation (15-20 minutes)

Practice Instructions:

1. Visualize your cells in renewal

2. Direct healing energy to areas of tension

3. Imagine telomeres strengthening

4. Generate feelings of youth and vitality

5. Hold this state with focused attention

Common Emotional-Biochemical Patterns

1. **The Stress Loop**

- Persistent worry thoughts

- Chronic muscle tension

- Elevated stress hormones

- Accelerated cellular aging

Breaking the Pattern:

- Mindful awareness of trigger thoughts

- Body-based stress release

- New response conditioning

- Regular relaxation practice

2. **The Trauma Hold**

- Stored emotional memory

- Physical armoring

- Inflammatory responses
- Compromised immune function

Breaking the Pattern:
- Gentle trauma-sensitive meditation
- Somatic release practices
- Building emotional safety
- Professional support when needed

3. **The Negativity Bias**
- Attention to problems
- Pessimistic thought patterns
- Stress chemistry activation
- Reduced repair capacity

Breaking the Pattern:
- Practicing gratitude
- Attention retraining
- Positive experience enrichment
- Building optimism circuits

Advanced Practices for Emotional Freedom

1. **The Quantum Pause**

This practice helps break the momentum of emotional habits by creating a gap between stimulus and response.

Instructions:
1. Notice emotional trigger
2. Take immediate conscious breath
3. Create 2-second pause
4. Choose new response
5. Reinforce new pattern

2. **Timeline Reimagining**

This practice helps release the emotional charge of past events

Instructions:
1. Identify limiting past experience
2. View it from observer perspective

3. Reimagine with new understanding

4. Generate healing emotion

5. Project new pattern forward

3. Future Self Integration

This practice helps create new emotional-biochemical patterns.

Instructions:

1. Visualize evolved future self

2. Feel their emotional state

3. Embody their perspective

4. Bridge to present moment

5. Live from new template

Creating New Cellular Conditions

The Biology of Transformation

When you break free from past conditioning, you create new biological conditions that support cellular health:

1. **Stress Response Reset**
   - Lowered baseline cortisol
   - Improved hormonal balance
   - Enhanced vagal tone
   - Better stress recovery

2. **Immune System Optimization**
   - Reduced inflammation
   - Improved immune function
   - Better cellular repair
   - Enhanced telomerase activity

3. **Gene Expression Shifts**
   - Activation of longevity genes
   - Reduced stress response genes
   - Enhanced repair mechanisms
   - Improved cellular resilience

Integration Practices for Daily Life

1. **Morning Pattern Break**
- 10-minute awareness practice
- Conscious emotional reset
- Setting daily intention
- Cellular renewal visualization

2. **Midday Reset**
- Quick body scan
- Emotional check-in
- Pattern interruption
- State optimization

3. **Evening Integration**
- Review daily patterns
- Release accumulated tension
- Generate healing states
- Set cellular renewal intention

Working with Challenging Patterns

1. **Deep-Seated Trauma**
- Start slowly and gently
- Build emotional safety
- Work with professional support
- Integrate somatic practices

2. **Resistant Patterns**
- Use gradual exposure
- Build resources first
- Layer new responses
- Celebrate small changes

3. **Complex Emotions**
- Parse component feelings
- Work with one aspect at a time
- Build emotional vocabulary
- Increase tolerance gradually

Signs of Progress

Physical Indicators

- Reduced muscle tension

- Better sleep quality

- Improved energy levels

- Enhanced immune function

Emotional Markers

- Greater emotional range

- Faster recovery from triggers

- Increased positive states

- Better stress resilience

Cognitive Shifts

- Reduced thought loops

- Enhanced perspective

- Improved concentration

- Greater mental clarity

Supporting Your Transformation

1. Environmental Factors

- Create supportive spaces

- Reduce unnecessary stress

- Build positive routines

- Optimize sleep environment

2. Relationship Patterns

- Communicate boundaries

- Seek supportive connections

- Release toxic relationships

- Build emotional safety

3. Lifestyle Practices

- Regular exercise

- Healthy nutrition

- Adequate rest

- Nature connection

The Path Forward: Living from New Patterns

Daily Implementation

1. Morning awareness practice
2. Regular pattern checks
3. Conscious response choices
4. Evening integration

Weekly Review

1. Pattern recognition
2. Progress assessment
3. Strategy adjustment
4. Practice refinement

Monthly Integration

1. Deep practice review
2. Pattern evolution tracking
3. Strategy updates
4. Future planning

Conclusion: From Past to Potential

Breaking free from past conditioning is not just about changing thoughts or behaviors—it's about creating new biological conditions that support cellular health and vitality. Through consistent practice and conscious awareness, you can transform limiting patterns into opportunities for growth and renewal.

Remember that this is a process of evolution, not revolution. Each time you notice and shift a pattern, you're creating new possibilities at the cellular level. Your body is incredibly responsive to change, and every new choice contributes to your cellular renewal.

In the next chapter, we'll explore how to cultivate positive expectancy—a powerful state that can enhance healing responses and support cellular regeneration.

Reflection Questions

1. What emotional patterns do you notice recurring in your life? How might these affect your cellular health?
2. Which practices resonate most strongly with you? How might you incorporate them into your daily routine?
3. What changes have you noticed since beginning to work with your patterns
4. How does understanding the biology of emotions influence your approach to personal growth?
5. What support systems might you need to sustain your transformation process?

6.Cultivating Positive Expectancy

Introduction

Positive expectancy is more than optimistic thinking—it's a powerful biological state that can influence health outcomes at the cellular level. As we explored in earlier chapters, beliefs and expectations create distinct biochemical environments within our bodies. When you genuinely expect healing or positive outcomes, your body often responds accordingly, activating repair mechanisms and optimizing cellular function.

This chapter explores how to cultivate positive expectancy through meditation and mindset practices, creating an internal environment that supports telomere maintenance and cellular renewal. We'll examine the science behind expectation's influence on biology and provide specific techniques to harness this power for healing and regeneration.

The Biology of Belief

The Biochemistry of Expectation

When you maintain positive expectations, your body responds with:

- Increased dopamine and serotonin production
- Reduced cortisol levels
- Enhanced immune system function
- Improved telomerase activity
- Optimized gene expression patterns

Research has shown that positive expectancy can:

1. Activate natural healing responses
2. Reduce inflammatory markers
3. Improve cellular repair mechanisms

4. Support telomere maintenance

5. Enhance stress resilience

The Expectancy-Biology Loop

How Expectations Shape Reality

Your expectations influence your biology through several pathways:

1. **Neural Pathways**
   - Activated reward circuits
   - Enhanced prefrontal function
   - Improved emotional regulation
   - Stronger mind-body connection

2. **Hormonal Cascades**
   - Balanced stress hormones
   - Increased growth factors
   - Optimized immune function
   - Enhanced cellular repair

3. **Genetic Expression**
   - Activated longevity genes
   - Reduced stress response genes
   - Improved cellular maintenance
   - Enhanced telomerase expression

Meditation Practices for Cultivating Positive Expectancy

1. **The Foundation Practice: Expectancy Meditation**

Basic Protocol (20-30 minutes)

1. **Preparation** (5 minutes)
   - Find a comfortable position
   - Ground your awareness in the body
   - Establish steady breathing
   - Set clear intention

2. **Body Activation** (10 minutes)
   - Scan body systematically
   - Notice areas of tension
   - Generate warmth and relaxation
   - Activate healing response

3. **Expectancy Generation** (10 minutes)
   - Visualize positive outcomes
   - Feel associated emotions
   - Engage multiple senses
   - Amplify positive sensations

4. **Integration** (5 minutes)
   - Anchor the experience
   - Set forward intention
   - Express gratitude
   - Close with affirmation

2. **The Cellular Optimization Practice**

Instructions for 20-minute practice:

1. **Cell Communication**
   - Direct attention to cellular level
   - Generate feelings of vitality
   - Visualize telomere strengthening
   - Feel cellular renewal

2. **Energy Activation**
   - Build subtle energy awareness
   - Direct healing intention
   - Amplify positive sensations
   - Maintain steady focus

3. **Integration**
   - Expand awareness throughout body
   - Feel systemic optimization
   - Set healing intention
   - Trust natural processes

Advanced Techniques for Deepening Practice

1. Quantum Field Meditation

Quantum field meditation, also known as Quantum Observation Meditation (QOM), draws parallels between quantum physics and the observer effect, suggesting that our conscious attention can influence our mental states and potentially shift our reality. It builds on the idea that at the quantum level, particles exist in multiple states (superposition) until observed, and proposes that our thoughts and emotions also exist in a similar state of potential until we consciously observe them[16].

Based on Dr. Joe Dispenza's work, this practice helps access expanded states of consciousness that support healing:

1. **Field Entry**
   - Release physical awareness
   - Enter quantum space
   - Feel infinite potential
   - Access universal energy

2. **Healing Activation**
   - Draw in vital force
   - Direct to needed areas
   - Feel cellular response
   - Trust deeper wisdom

3. **Reality Creation**
   - Envision desired outcome
   - Feel it as present now
   - Generate gratitude
   - Maintain coherent state

2. Timeline Integration Practice

---

[16] *Yupapin, Preecha & Punthawanunt, Suphanchai. (2016). Quantum Meditation: The Self-Spirit Projection. International Journal of Philosophy Study. 4. 5. 10.14355/ijps.2016.04.002.*

This technique helps align past, present, and future with positive expectancy:

1. **Past Resolution**
   - Review limiting experiences
   - Release old patterns
   - Reframe with wisdom
   - Find hidden gifts
2. **Present Activation**
   - Feel current potential
   - Generate optimal state
   - Trust natural healing
   - Embrace uncertainty
3. **Future Bridge**
   - Connect to future self
   - Feel accomplished healing
   - Bridge to present moment
   - Live from new template

Scientific Research Supporting Positive Expectancy

Key Studies and Findings

1. **Placebo Response Research**

Placebo response research examines the effects of seemingly inactive treatments, like inert pills or sham surgeries, on patient health and well-being in clinical trials. It's crucial for understanding how expectations, beliefs, and other psychological factors influence treatment outcomes and for distinguishing true treatment effects from the influence of the placebo effect[17].

---

[17] *Munnangi S, Sundjaja JH, Singh K, et al. Placebo Effect. [Updated 2023 Nov 13]. In: StatPearls [Internet]. Treasure Island (FL): StatPearls Publishing; 2025 Jan-. Available from: https://www.ncbi.nlm.nih.gov/books/NBK513296/*

Following effects are observed under the Placebo effect in targetted person:

- Activation of endogenous opioids
- Enhanced immune function
- Reduced inflammation
- Improved healing rates

2. **Meditation Effects**

- Increased telomerase activity
- Better stress regulation
- Enhanced gene expression
- Improved cellular repair

3. **Mind-Body Connection**

- Nervous system optimization
- Hormonal balance
- Improved cellular function
- Enhanced healing response

Integration Practices for Daily Life

1. **Morning Priming Protocol**

10-minute morning practice:

1. Set positive intention
2. Generate healing state
3. Visualize optimal health
4. Feel gratitude and trust

2. **Midday Reset**

5-minute practice:

1. Quick body scan
2. Release tension
3. Renew expectancy
4. Reset intention

3. **Evening Integration**

15-minute practice:

1. Review daily experiences
2. Release limiting patterns
3. Generate healing state
4. Set overnight intention

Working with Challenges

1. **Dealing with Doubt**
- Notice doubt arising
- Accept without judgment
- Return to positive focus
- Build evidence base

2. **Managing Setbacks**
- Maintain broader perspective
- Learn from experience
- Adjust approach as needed
- Keep fundamental trust

3. **Sustaining Practice**
- Build regular routine
- Create support system
- Track progress
- Celebrate small wins

Creating Supportive Conditions

1. **Environmental Factors**
- Optimize physical space
- Reduce negative influences
- Create healing atmosphere
- Support natural rhythms

2. **Relationship Dynamics**
- Communicate needs clearly
- Build supportive connections
- Release toxic relationships
- Share positive intentions

3. **Lifestyle Practices**

- Align daily activities
- Support cellular health
- Maintain energy balance
- Foster natural healing

Measuring Progress

1. Subjective Indicators

- Improved mood
- Better sleep
- Enhanced energy
- Greater resilience

2. Objective Markers

- Reduced inflammation
- Better immune function
- Improved recovery
- Enhanced vitality

3. Practice Developments

- Deeper meditation
- Stronger focus
- Clear intention
- Sustained trust

Advanced Concepts and Applications

1. Field Theory and Healing

Field theory in healing suggests that individuals are not isolated entities but are part of a larger interconnected system, or "field," that influences their well-being. This field can be understood as a network of relationships, environments, and even consciousness, affecting an individual's physical, emotional, and spiritual state. By understanding and interacting with this field, individuals can promote healing and growth[18].

---

[18] *The Healing Field: Energy, Consciousness and Transformation by Peter Mark Adams*

- Understanding quantum effects
- Accessing unified field
- Working with energy
- Amplifying intention

2. Consciousness and Cells

The idea that cells themselves possess a form of consciousness is a controversial, yet evolving, topic. Some scientists and philosophers propose that consciousness may be a fundamental property of life, emerging with the first cells, while others maintain that consciousness is a complex phenomenon primarily associated with higher organisms like humans and animals[19].

- Direct communication
- Energy transmission
- Information flow
- Coherent states

Conclusion: The Power of Positive Expectancy

Cultivating positive expectancy is not about denying reality or maintaining superficial positivity. It's about creating an internal environment that supports natural healing processes and optimal cellular function. Through consistent practice and deep understanding, you can develop this capacity as a powerful tool for health and renewal.

Remember that each moment of practice contributes to your cellular health and overall wellbeing. Trust in your body's innate wisdom while maintaining the positive expectancy that supports its optimal function.

In the next chapter, we'll explore how stress affects telomeres and discover specific meditation techniques to manage stress response for better cellular health.

---

https://amzn.in/d/8cVZTxY
[19] *https://www.embopress.org/doi/full/10.1038/s44319-024-00127-4*

Reflection Questions

1. How has your relationship with expectancy changed through these practices?

2. What challenges have you encountered in maintaining positive expectancy?

3. Which practices resonate most strongly with your experience?

4. How might you deepen your practice in daily life?

5. What support do you need to maintain consistent practice?

Practice Guidelines

1. Start with basic protocols

2. Build gradually and consistently

3. Trust your experience

4. Maintain regular practice

5. Seek support when needed

7.Stress, Telomeres, and the Meditative Solution

Introduction

Stress is not just a psychological experience—it's a complex biological cascade that can directly impact your cellular health and aging process. Research by Dr. Elizabeth Blackburn and Dr. Elissa Epel has shown that chronic stress is one of the most significant factors in telomere shortening. However, the same research reveals that how we respond to stress may be more important than the stressors themselves.

This chapter explores the intricate relationship between stress and telomere biology, and provides specific meditation techniques to transform your stress response. By understanding and working skillfully with stress, you can create conditions that support rather than undermine cellular health.

The Biology of Stress

Acute vs. Chronic Stress

Acute Stress Response:

- Temporary cortisol elevation

- Enhanced immune function

- Improved focus and alertness

- Quick recovery to baseline

Chronic Stress Pattern:

- Persistent cortisol elevation

- Compromised immune function

- Accelerated telomere shortening

- Reduced cellular repair

Stress Response Pathways

1. **HPA Axis Activation**
   - Hypothalamic signaling
   - Pituitary hormone release
   - Adrenal cortisol production
   - Systemic effects

2. **Sympathetic Nervous System**
   - Adrenaline release
   - Increased heart rate
   - Blood pressure elevation
   - Energy mobilization

3. **Cellular Impact**
   - Oxidative stress increase
   - DNA damage potential
   - Telomere erosion
   - Reduced repair capacity

Telomeres and Stress: The Connection

Direct Effects

1. **Oxidative Damage**
   - Free radical production
   - DNA strand breaks
   - Telomere vulnerability
   - Accelerated shortening

2. **Inflammatory Response**
   - Cytokine elevation
   - Chronic inflammation
   - Cellular aging
   - Reduced telomerase

Indirect Effects

1. **Behavioral Changes**

- Poor sleep quality
- Dietary choices
- Reduced exercise
- Social isolation

2. **Mental Patterns**
   - Rumination
   - Worry cycles
   - Negative thinking
   - Emotional reactivity

The Meditation Solution

Basic Stress Response Protocol

20-Minute Practice:

1. Recognition Phase (5 minutes)
   - Notice stress signals
   - Locate bodily tension
   - Identify thought patterns
   - Observe emotional state

2. Release Phase (5 minutes)
   - Conscious breathing
   - Progressive relaxation
   - Mental clearing
   - Emotional release

3. Reset Phase (5 minutes)
   - Activate parasympathetic
   - Generate calm state
   - Set new intention
   - Feel cellular renewal

4. Integration Phase (5 minutes)
   - Anchor new state
   - Strengthen resilience
   - Build positive expectancy

- Trust natural healing

Advanced Stress Transformation Practices

1. Quantum Coherence Meditation

Quantum coherence meditation is a practice that aims to harmonize the mind, body, and spirit by leveraging principles of quantum physics. It involves cultivating a state of internal coherence, where different parts of the brain and body function in sync, much like the coordinated behavior of quantum particles[20].

30-Minute Protocol:

- Enter coherent state

- Access unified field

- Direct healing intention

- Maintain elevated state

2. Cellular Stress Release

25-Minute Protocol:

- Connect with cells

- Release stored stress

- Activate telomerase

- Support renewal

3. Time-Space Medicine

35-Minute Protocol:

- Transcend linear time

- Access healing potential

- Bridge to health state

- Collapse old patterns

Scientific Evidence and Research

Key Studies on Stress and Telomeres

1. **Blackburn-Epel Research**

---

[20] *https://insighttimer.com/drsukhi/guided-meditations/coherence-meditation*

Blackburn-Epel research[21] focuses on telomeres, protective caps at the ends of chromosomes that shorten with age. Their work, particularly with Elissa Epel, has highlighted the impact of stress, particularly chronic stress, on telomere maintenance and length. They've demonstrated that chronic stress can lead to shorter telomeres and potentially accelerate the aging process. Following aspects have been focused on and adverse impact of stress established:

- Stress-telomere correlation
- Biological aging markers
- Intervention effects
- Long-term outcomes

2. Meditation Impact Studies

Meditation practice has been linked to increased telomere length, potentially slowing down the cellular aging process. Studies suggest that meditation reduces stress and inflammation, which can contribute to telomere shortening. Some research indicates that meditation, particularly loving-kindness meditation, may increase telomerase activity, an enzyme that helps maintain telomere length[22].

Following positive aspects have emerged from these studies:

- Telomerase activation
- Stress reduction
- Cellular repair
- Gene expression

---

[21] *https://www.ucsf.edu/news/2011/02/103672/aging-chronic-disease-and-telomeres-are-linked-recent-studies*

[22] *Schutte NS, Malouff JM, Keng SL. Meditation and telomere length: a meta-analysis. Psychol Health. 2020 Aug;35(8):901-915. doi: 10.1080/08870446.2019.1707827. Epub 2020 Jan 5. PMID: 31903785.*

3. Mind-Body Integration

Mind-body integration research explores the bidirectional influence between mental and physical states, demonstrating how thoughts, emotions, and behaviors impact bodily functions, and vice versa. Studies in this field examine how stress, for example, can trigger biochemical responses affecting the immune system, heart rate, and other bodily processes. Conversely, physical conditions like chronic illnesses can influence mood, anxiety, and cognitive function[23].

Following areas are found relevant in these studies:

- Nervous system effects
- Hormonal balance
- Immune function
- Cellular health

Daily Integration Practices

1. Morning Stress Prevention

10-Minute Protocol:
1. Set positive intention
2. Generate coherent state
3. Prepare for challenges
4. Build stress resilience

2. Midday Reset

5-Minute Protocol:

---

[23] Brower V. Mind-body research moves towards the mainstream. EMBO Rep. 2006 Apr;7(4):358-61. doi: 10.1038/sj.embor.7400671. PMID: 16585935; PMCID: PMC1456909.

1. Quick stress scan
2. Release tension
3. Reset nervous system
4. Return to balance

3. Evening Integration

15-Minute Protocol:
1. Release accumulated stress
2. Process daily experiences
3. Activate renewal
4. Prepare for rest

Working with Specific Stressors

1. Work-Related Stress

Management Techniques:
- Boundary setting
- Time management
- Energy optimization
- Response choice

2. Relationship Stress

Transformation Practices:
- Communication skills
- Emotional regulation
- Boundary maintenance
- Energy protection

3. Health-Related Stress

Coping Strategies:
- Uncertainty management
- Treatment support
- Healing activation
- Trust building

Advanced Concepts in Stress Transformation

1. The Quantum Perspective

A "quantum perspective" on mental stress transformation refers to applying concepts from quantum physics to understand and potentially manage mental stress. This approach often explores the idea that the brain, like a quantum system, can exist in multiple states simultaneously and that conscious observation can affect these states. By drawing parallels between quantum phenomena like superposition and entanglement and mental states, it suggests that we can actively influence our emotional and cognitive experiences through techniques like meditation and by reframing our perceptions of stressors[24].

Understanding stress through quantum biology entails following aspects:
- Field effects
- Non-local healing
- Information transfer
- Coherent states

---

[24] *https://en.wikipedia.org/wiki/Quantum_mind#:~:text=The%20quantum%20mind%20or%20quantum,entanglement%20and%20superposition%20that%20cause use*

2. Epigenetic Influences

Meditation may influence gene expression through epigenetic mechanisms, affecting various biological processes and potentially impacting well-being. Specifically, meditation practices like mindfulness, Vipassana, Yoga, and Tai Chi have been linked to changes in epigenetic markers such as DNA methylation, chromatin components, and microRNAs. These changes may contribute to reduced stress, improved mood, and enhanced resilience[25].

How meditation affects gene expression:
- Stress response genes
- Repair mechanisms
- Longevity factors
- Cellular optimization

3. Consciousness and Healing

The role of awareness in stress transformation:
- Observer state
- Choice point
- Response flexibility
- Elevated consciousness

Creating Sustainable Change

1. Environmental Optimization
- Stress-free spaces
- Support systems

---

[25] Verdone L, Caserta M, Ben-Soussan TD, Venditti S. *On the road to resilience: Epigenetic effects of meditation. Vitam Horm. 2023;122:339-376. doi: 10.1016/bs.vh.2022.12.009. Epub 2023 Feb 10. PMID: 36863800.*

- Natural elements
- Healing atmosphere

2. Relationship Dynamics

- Clear communication
- Healthy boundaries
- Supportive connections
- Energy management

3. Lifestyle Integration

- Regular practice
- Healthy routines
- Sleep optimization
- Nutrition support

Measuring Progress

1. Subjective Indicators

- Stress perception
- Recovery speed
- Emotional balance
- Overall wellbeing

2. Objective Markers

- Heart rate variability
- Sleep quality
- Energy levels

- Physical symptoms

3. Practice Development

- Meditation depth
- Response flexibility
- Stress resilience
- Healing capacity

The Path Forward

1. Continuous Development

- Regular practice
- Skill building
- Understanding deepening
- Experience integration

2. Challenge Management

- Pattern recognition
- Response choice
- Recovery optimization
- Learning integration

3. Long-term Vision

- Health promotion
- Cellular optimization
- Consciousness evolution
- Continued growth

Conclusion: From Stress to Strength

Understanding the relationship between stress and telomere biology empowers you to make choices that support cellular health. Through consistent meditation practice and conscious stress transformation, you can create an internal environment that promotes telomere maintenance and overall wellbeing.

Remember that each moment of practice contributes to your resilience and cellular health. Trust in your body's capacity for renewal while maintaining the practices that support its optimal function.

In the next chapter, we'll explore meditation practices specifically designed to influence genetic expression, further enhancing your capacity for cellular renewal.

Reflection Questions

1. How has your understanding of stress changed through these practices?

2. Which techniques have been most effective for your stress transformation?

3. What challenges remain in your stress management practice?

4. How might you deepen your practice for greater resilience?

5. What support do you need to maintain consistent practice?

Practice Guidelines

1. Start with basic protocols
2. Build gradually and consistently
3. Trust your experience
4. Maintain regular practice
5. Seek support when needed

PART III

THE PRACTICE

7.Meditation for Genetic Expression

Introduction

The discovery that gene expression can be influenced by our thoughts, emotions, and behaviors represents a revolutionary understanding in biology. This field, known as epigenetics, reveals that while we cannot change our genetic code, we can influence how our genes are read and expressed. Meditation, as research increasingly shows, can be a powerful tool for optimizing genetic expression, particularly for genes involved in stress response, inflammation, and cellular aging.

This chapter explores specific meditation practices designed to influence genetic expression, with a particular focus on genes related to telomerase activity and cellular renewal. By understanding and working with these mechanisms, you can actively participate in your cellular health optimization.

Epigenetics, in simple terms, refers to how your environment and lifestyle choices can influence how your genes function, without changing the genes themselves. Meditation, a mindful practice, can be seen as an environmental factor that can lead to epigenetic changes, potentially affecting your health and well-being[26].

---

[26] *Molecules of Silence: Effects of Meditation on Gene Expression and Epigenetics, Venditti Sabrina , Verdone Loredana , Reale Anna , Vetriani Valerio , Caserta Micaela , Zampieri Michele, Frontiers in Psychology, Volume 11 – 2020,*

What is Epigenetics?

- **Not DNA mutations:** Epigenetic changes don't alter the DNA sequence (the "code" of life).

- **Like a switch:** They act like switches, turning genes on or off, or changing how they are used.

- **Reversible:** These changes can be reversed, meaning they are not permanent.

- **Influenced by environment:** Epigenetic changes can be triggered by various factors, including stress, diet, and lifestyle.

How Meditation Impacts Epigenetics

- **Stress reduction:**

  Meditation, especially mindfulness-based practices, can help reduce stress levels.

- **Gene expression changes:**

  Some studies suggest that meditation may alter the expression of genes involved in stress response, inflammation, and immune function.

- **Increased resilience:**

  By modulating the epigenetic landscape, meditation may contribute to increased resilience to stress and improved well-being.

- **Mind-body connection:**

---

https://www.frontiersin.org/journals/psychology/articles/10.3389/fpsyg.2020.01767, doi:10.3389/fpsyg.2020.01767

The brain and body are interconnected, and meditation can influence physiological processes at the molecular level, including epigenetic mechanisms.

Examples of Epigenetic Effects of Meditation

- **Inflammation:**

  Meditation practices like yoga have been shown to positively influence the expression of genes related to inflammation in certain conditions.

- **Stress response:**

  Meditation may reduce the activation of genes related to stress responses, like the HPA axis.

- **Improved physical recovery:**

  Studies indicate that mindfulness practice can lead to changes in gene expression that contribute to faster physical recovery from stressful situations.

- **Changes in brain waves:**

  Meditation may increase alpha and theta brain waves, which are associated with relaxation and mindfulness, potentially impacting gene expression.

In essence, meditation can be seen as a tool for influencing epigenetics, offering a potential path to enhance resilience, reduce stress, and promote overall well-being through the power of the mind and its influence on gene activity.

Key Genes Affected by Meditation

1. **Stress Response Genes**
   - Cortisol regulation
   - Inflammatory pathways

- Oxidative stress
- Recovery mechanisms

2. **Longevity Genes**
   - Telomerase expression
   - Cellular repair
   - Anti-aging factors
   - Protective elements

3. **Immune Function Genes**
   - Inflammatory markers
   - Immune regulation
   - Recovery processes
   - Cellular protection

Meditation Practices for Genetic Optimization

1. **Foundation Practice: Genetic Expression Meditation**

30-Minute Protocol:

1. Preparation (5 minutes)
   - Comfortable position
   - Breathing awareness
   - Body grounding
   - Intention setting

2. Gene Activation (10 minutes)
   - Cellular awareness
   - Energy cultivation
   - Healing intention
   - Expression optimization

3. Integration (10 minutes)
   - System-wide integration
   - Pattern reinforcement
   - State anchoring
   - Future pacing

4. Completion (5 minutes)
   - Gratitude generation
   - Practice closure
   - State maintenance
   - Forward intention

2. **Advanced DNA Meditation**

45-Minute Protocol:

1. **DNA Connection**
   - Visualize double helix
   - Feel cellular presence
   - Access genetic wisdom
   - Direct healing intention

2. **Expression Optimization**
   - Target specific genes
   - Activate beneficial expression
   - Suppress harmful patterns
   - Enhance repair mechanisms

3. **Field Integration**
   - Access quantum field
   - Draw healing energy

- Direct to DNA
- Maintain coherence

Scientific Research Support

Key Studies

1. Meditation Effects on Gene Expression
- Inflammatory reduction
- Stress response improvement
- Telomerase activation
- Cellular repair enhancement

2. Epigenetic Changes

Epigenetic changes[27] are heritable alterations in gene expression that occur without changes to the DNA sequence itself. These changes can be caused by modifications to DNA and its associated proteins, impacting how genes are read and utilized. They can be influenced by various factors, including age, diet, stress, and disease.
- Methylation patterns
- Histone modifications
- RNA regulation
- Long-term effects

3. Clinical Outcomes
- Health improvements
- Aging markers
- Disease prevention

---

[27] Al Aboud NM, Tupper C, Jialal I. Genetics, Epigenetic Mechanism. [Updated 2023 Aug 14]. In: StatPearls [Internet]. Treasure Island (FL): StatPearls Publishing; 2025 Jan-. Available from: https://www.ncbi.nlm.nih.gov/books/NBK532999/

- Recovery enhancement

Practical Applications

Daily Practice Integration

1. Morning Protocol
- Gene activation
- Expression optimization
- State setting
- Intention reinforcement

2. Midday Reset
- Quick recalibration
- Pattern reinforcement
- Energy renewal
- Focus restoration

3. Evening Integration
- Day processing
- Pattern optimization
- Repair activation
- Renewal preparation

Working with Specific Conditions

1. Stress-Related Issues
- Cortisol regulation
- Anxiety reduction
- Recovery enhancement
- Resilience building

2. Inflammatory Conditions
- Anti-inflammatory activation
- Immune balancing
- Pain management
- Healing support

3. Aging Concerns
- Telomerase activation
- Repair enhancement
- Renewal stimulation
- Vitality increase

Advanced Concepts

Quantum Biology Perspectives

Quantum biology[28] investigates how quantum mechanics principles apply to biological processes, particularly those that cannot be adequately explained by classical physics. It explores phenomena like quantum coherence, tunneling, and entanglement in biological systems, focusing on processes like photosynthesis, enzyme catalysis, avian navigation, and olfaction.
- Field effects on DNA
- Non-local influence
- Information transfer
- Coherence states

---

[28] *Eissa ME. Quantum biology from theory to the future of medicine and pharmacy: A review on a revolutionary change in our perception of life. Universal Journal of Pharmaceutical Research 2024; 9(5): 113-121. http://doi.org/10.22270/ujpr.v9i5.1199*

Creating Supportive Conditions

1. Environmental Factors

- Practice space
- Energy quality
- Natural elements
- Support systems

2. Lifestyle Integration

- Daily routines
- Nutrition support
- Movement practices
- Rest patterns

3. Relationship Dynamics

- Support network
- Communication patterns
- Energy management
- Boundary maintenance

Measuring Progress

1. Subjective Markers

- Energy levels
- Sleep quality
- Emotional balance
- Overall wellbeing

2. Objective Indicators

- Health markers
- Recovery rates
- Performance measures
- Aging indicators

3. Practice Development

- Meditation depth
- Understanding growth
- Technique refinement
- Experience integration

Conclusion: Activating Your Genetic Potential

Understanding how meditation can influence genetic expression opens new possibilities for health and healing. Through consistent practice and conscious engagement, you can create conditions that optimize your genetic potential and support cellular health.

Remember that each meditation session is an opportunity to influence your genetic expression positively. Trust in your body's innate wisdom while maintaining the practices that support its optimal function.

In the next chapter, we'll explore the emotional connection to cellular health and how specific meditation practices can help create beneficial emotional states.

Reflection Questions

1. How has your understanding of genetic influence changed through these practices?

2. Which techniques resonate most strongly with your experience?

3. What challenges have you encountered in your practice?

4. How might you deepen your engagement with these practices?

5. What support do you need to maintain consistent practice?

Practice Guidelines

1. Start with basic protocols
2. Build gradually and consistently
3. Trust your experience
4. Maintain regular practice
5. Seek support when needed

9. The Emotional Connection

Introduction

Emotions are not just abstract feelings—they are biological events that create specific chemical signatures in your body. Each emotional state triggers a cascade of hormones, neurotransmitters, and other signaling molecules that can either support or undermine cellular health. Research has shown that emotional states can directly influence telomere length and telomerase activity, making emotional regulation a crucial aspect of cellular health.

Dr. Elizabeth Blackburn's research demonstrates that chronic negative emotions accelerate telomere shortening, while positive emotional states can support telomere maintenance. Understanding and working skillfully with emotions through meditation becomes a powerful tool for influencing cellular aging and renewal.

The Biology of Emotions

Emotional Biochemistry

1. **Positive Emotions**
   - Increased DHEA

Dehydroepiandrosterone (DHEA) is a hormone that your body naturally produces in the adrenal gland. DHEA helps produce other hormones, including testosterone and estrogen. Natural

DHEA levels peak in early adulthood and then slowly fall as you age.

 - Balanced cortisol

Cortisol is a steroid hormone, commonly called the "stress hormone," produced by the adrenal glands. It plays a crucial role in the body's response to stress, influencing various physiological processes and impacting numerous organs.

 - Enhanced oxytocin

Oxytocin is a hormone and neuropeptide produced in the hypothalamus and released by the posterior pituitary gland. It plays a crucial role in various behaviors, including social bonding, love, reproduction, childbirth, and the postpartum period. In addition to its influence on social behavior, oxytocin also stimulates uterine contractions during labor and milk ejection during breastfeeding.

 - Optimal immune function

2. Negative Emotions
 - Elevated cortisol
 - Increased inflammation
 - Reduced repair capacity
 - Accelerated aging

Cellular Impact of Emotions

1. Direct Effects
 - Gene expression changes
 - Telomerase activity
 - Inflammatory markers
 - Cellular repair rates

2. Indirect Effects

- Behavioral changes
- Sleep patterns
- Eating habits
- Social connections

Core Emotional Regulation Practices

1. Foundation Practice: Emotional Awareness Meditation

30-Minute Protocol:

1. Preparation (5 minutes)
   - Comfortable posture
   - Breathing awareness
   - Body grounding
   - Open attention

2. Emotional Scanning (10 minutes)
   - Notice feelings
   - Track sensations
   - Observe patterns
   - Stay present

3. Integration (10 minutes)
   - Process emotions
   - Release tension
   - Generate balance
   - Build resilience

4. Completion (5 minutes)
   - State anchoring
   - Future pacing

- Gratitude practice
- Gentle closure

2. **Heart Coherence Meditation**

Heart coherence is a state where the heart, mind, and emotions align, creating a harmonious and balanced rhythm. It occurs when the heart's rhythms become smooth and ordered.

25-Minute Protocol:

1. Heart Connection
   - Focus attention
   - Feel heartbeat
   - Generate appreciation
   - Build coherence

2. Emotional Optimization
   - Amplify positive states
   - Transform challenging emotions
   - Maintain balance
   - Enhance resilience

3. Cellular Integration
   - Connect heart-cell communication
   - Direct coherent energy
   - Support telomere health
   - Enhance repair

Practical Applications for Daily Life

1. Morning Emotional Attunement

10-Minute Protocol:

1. Check-in
   - Emotional awareness
   - Body scanning
   - Energy assessment
   - Intention setting

2. Regulation
   - Balance emotions
   - Generate coherence
   - Set positive state
   - Anchor experience

2. Midday Reset

5-Minute Protocol:
1. Quick Assessment
   - Emotional check
   - Energy reset
   - State optimization
   - Pattern adjustment

2. Integration
   - Release tension
   - Restore balance
   - Renew energy
   - Reset intention

3. Evening Integration

15-Minute Protocol:
1. Day Review
   - Process emotions

- Release patterns
- Find learning
- Create closure

2. Preparation
   - Set healing state
   - Activate renewal
   - Generate peace
   - Support rest

Conclusion: Emotions as Healing Tools

Understanding the profound connection between emotions and cellular health opens new possibilities for conscious healing. Through consistent practice and emotional awareness, you can create internal conditions that support telomere maintenance and cellular renewal.

Remember that each emotion offers an opportunity for growth and healing. By working skillfully with your emotional landscape, you create an internal environment that supports optimal cellular function and overall wellbeing.

In the next chapter, we'll explore living in the quantum field and how accessing expanded states of consciousness can enhance cellular healing and regeneration.

Reflection Questions

1. How has your relationship with emotions evolved through these practices?

2. Which techniques have been most effective for your emotional regulation?

3. What patterns have you noticed in your emotional landscape?

4. How might you deepen your emotional awareness practice?

5. What support do you need to maintain emotional balance?

Practice Guidelines

1. Start with basic awareness
2. Build regulation skills gradually
3. Trust your experience
4. Maintain consistent practice
5. Seek support when needed

10.Living in the Quantum Field

Introduction

The quantum field represents the underlying fabric of reality where everything is interconnected and consciousness plays a fundamental role. Dr. Joe Dispenza's work demonstrates how accessing this field through meditation can create profound changes in biology and consciousness. When we understand how to access and work with the quantum field, we open new possibilities for healing and cellular regeneration.

This chapter explores practical methods for accessing expanded states of consciousness that can influence cellular health, telomere maintenance, and overall wellbeing. By combining ancient wisdom with modern quantum understanding, we create a powerful approach to transformation.

Understanding the Quantum Field

The idea of a "Quantum Field" within the context of self-healing is a fascinating intersection of physics and the human experience. It suggests that our thoughts, emotions, and intentions, which are ultimately energy in a quantum sense, can influence our physical health. This idea is often explored through techniques like meditation and visualization, which aim to harness the power of our inner energy to promote wellbeing. While not yet mainstream scientific understanding, it is an area of active research and exploration.

Fundamental Concepts

1. Field Properties
   - Non-locality
   - Interconnectedness
   - Potentiality
   - Observer effect

2. Consciousness Impact
   - Intention influence
   - Information transfer
   - Reality creation
   - Healing potential

3. Biological Interface
   - Cell communication
   - Energy transmission
   - Information flow
   - System coherence

Core Quantum Field Practices

1. **Foundation Practice: Quantum Field Access**

45-Minute Protocol:

1. Preparation (10 minutes)
   - Physical relaxation
   - Energy awareness
   - Consciousness expansion
   - Field connection

2. Field Immersion (20 minutes)
   - Release physical awareness
   - Access quantum space
   - Feel infinite potential
   - Direct healing intention

3. Integration (10 minutes)
   - System coherence
   - Pattern establishment
   - Reality creation
   - Future bridging

4. Completion (5 minutes)
   - Gentle return
   - State anchoring
   - Physical grounding
   - Integration setting

2. Advanced Quantum Healing

60-Minute Protocol:

1. Field Entry
   - Consciousness expansion
   - Energy elevation
   - Dimension access
   - Potential activation

2. Healing Activation
   - Information access
   - Energy direction
   - Pattern transformation

- System optimization

3. Reality Creation
   - Future visualization
   - State generation
   - Pattern establishment
   - Integration process

Conclusion: Living in Quantum Reality

Understanding and working with the quantum field opens unprecedented possibilities for healing and transformation. Through consistent practice and conscious engagement, you can access states of consciousness that support optimal cellular function and overall wellbeing.

Remember that you are always connected to the quantum field—these practices simply help you access and work with it consciously. Trust in your ability to create positive change while maintaining the practices that support your evolution.

In the next chapter, we'll explore Patanjali Yoga Sutra to develop a philosophical understanding of meditation process.

Reflection Questions

1. How has your understanding of reality shifted through quantum field practice?

2. Which techniques have been most effective for your field connection?

3. What changes have you noticed in your life through these practices?

4. How might you deepen your quantum field engagement?

5. What support do you need to maintain consistent practice?

Practice Guidelines

1. Start with basic protocols
2. Build gradually and consistently
3. Trust your experience
4. Maintain regular practice
5. Seek support when needed

PART IV

PHILOSOPHY OF MEDITATION

11. Patanjali Yoga Sutra

Introduction

Meditation is key process in this book. While many simple guides have been described in earlier chapter to achieve limited objective of good health and stress reduction, it is important to understand philosophical underpinnings of meditation through an authentic source in Hindu scriptures.

In Hindu thoughts , Patanjali yoga sutra[29] is considered to be one structured approach towards realization of our true self. As a departure from the philosophical theories, it attempts to provide us a stage by stage blueprint for action.

No affiliation with any religion is necessary. Any person interested in this self discovery journey can get on board. However, there are essential steps that need to be taken. These are universal in nature and there cannot be any short cut.

According to Patanjali, the key goal of the journey is to still (calm down) our mental tendencies (Chitta Vrati) . When our highest mind layer called 'Chitta' is perfectly still with no tendencies perturbing it, one gets a realization of one's true self.

It is akin to viewing the image of a full moon in the calm water of a lake. The lake is like our Chitta and viewing the moon is the process of self realization.

---

[29] *https://www.yogapradipika.com/yoga-sutra*

This process of stilling or calming the Chitta and viewing our true self can only be understood by undertaking the journey.

As our mental faculties are already dropped on the way towards the final goal of self realization (Samadhi), it is impossible to describe it by a realized seeker. Words fail him; so to say. It can only be alluded to and hence guidance by a suitable teacher is recommended.

However, it is a very personal , life changing experience that alters our self image permanently and one goes through life after this self realization, with equanimity under pleasure and pain.

The Yoga Sutras of Patanjali provide a comprehensive blueprint for self-realization and spiritual enlightenment. The main purpose of yoga is to learn to control our mind and not be controlled by our thoughts. Through yoga we learn to dissociate from our thoughts.

The teachings and practices of the Yoga Sutras are based on three principles:
1) Suffering is not caused by forces outside of us but by our faulty and limited perception of life and of who we are. Suffering is not caused by the situation, but by our thoughts about the situation.
2) The unwavering peace we seek is realized by experiencing the unlimited and eternal peace that is our true identity. Though hidden by our ignorance, it exists within us, waiting to be revealed. Peace exists within us.
3) Peace and self-realization is attained by mastering the mind. Only a single-pointed, calm mind can reveal the true self.

There are 196 sutras (aphorisms) presented in four chapters (or padas). Each pada emphasizes a different aspect of the science of yoga.

Patanjali divided his Yoga Sutras into 4 chapters or books (Sanskrit pada), containing in all 196 aphorisms (Sutras), divided as follows:

Pada 1: Concentration (Samadhi Pada)

Pada 2: Practice (Sadhana Pada)

Pada 3: Experiences (Vibhuti Pada)

Pada 4: Absolute Freedom (Kaivalya Pada)

The Eight Limbs of Yoga (Ashtanga Yoga):

The Yoga Sutras outline an eight-fold path known as Ashtanga Yoga, which serves as a systematic approach to self-realization.

Figure 1 describes the hierarchy of these limbs. The end objective of Samadhi or Self Realization is achieved only after the remaining seven underlying stages are firmly established.

Yama and Niyam are the foundational attributes and are at the same level. Similarly Asan and Pranayama are shown at same level as they relate to our body.

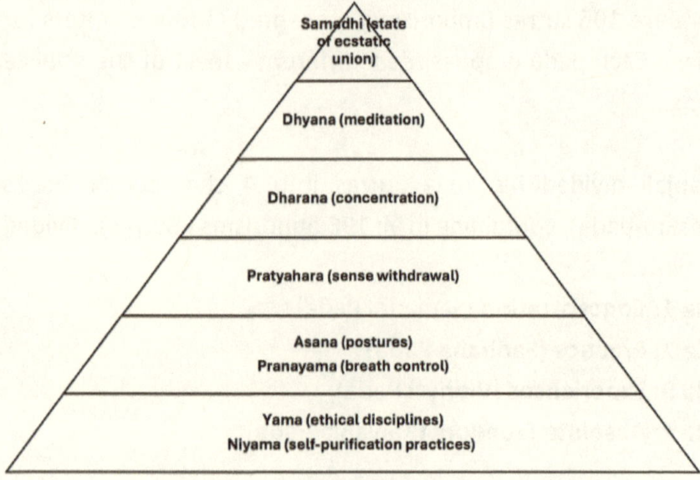

Figure 1: Hierarchy of Eight Limbs of Yoga

These eight limbs are as given below:

Yama (ethical disciplines)

- Ahimsa (non-violence)

- Satya (truthfulness)

- Asteya (non-stealing)

- Brahmacharya (moderation of the senses/right use of energy)

- Aparigraha (non-greed)

Niyama (self-purification practices)

- Saucha (cleanliness) Saucha can be translated as 'cleanliness', but it doesn't just mean physical cleanliness

- Santosha (contentment)

- Tapas (discipline)

- Svadhyaya (self study)

- Isvara Pranidhana (surrendering to a higher power)

Asana (postures)
Pranayama (breath control)
Pratyahara (sense withdrawal)
Dharana (concentration)
Dhyana (meditation)
Samadhi (state of ecstatic union)

Stilling the Modifications of the Mind:
A central tenet of the Yoga Sutras is that the goal is to stop (still) the fluctuations of the mind (chitta vritti nirodhah). By quieting the constant chatter and distractions of the mind, one can experience the true nature of the Self or Purusha.

The Practice of Kriya Yoga:
Patanjali outlines a three-part process called Kriya Yoga, which consists of tapas (austerity/discipline), svadhyaya (self-study), and Ishvara pranidhana (surrender to the Divine). This practice purifies the body, mind, and spirit, preparing the individual for self-realization.

The Contemplation of Ishvara (The Lord):
The Yoga Sutras recommend the contemplation of Ishvara, or the Lord, as a means to attain the highest form of Samadhi (union). This can be achieved through devotion, repetition of sacred words (mantras), or contemplation on the qualities of the Divine.

The Removal of Afflictions (Kleshas):
Patanjali identifies five afflictions (kleshas) that hinder self-realization: ignorance (avidya), egoism (asmita), attachment

(raga), aversion (dvesha), and clinging to life (abhinivesha). The Yoga Sutras provide methods to overcome these obstacles.

The Development of Discriminative Discernment (Viveka Khyati):

Viveka Khyati, or discriminative discernment, is the ability to distinguish between the eternal Purusha (Self) and the temporary Prakriti (material world). This insight is essential for self-realization.

By systematically following the eight limbs, practicing Kriya Yoga, contemplating the Divine, removing afflictions, and developing discriminative discernment, the Yoga Sutras of Patanjali provide a comprehensive framework for attaining the ultimate goal of self-realization and union with the Divine.

It may be observed that the first five limbs starting from Yama/Niyamas upto Pratyahara (sense withdrawal)or the Kriya yoga are focussing on external part of the seeker's personality.However, without this tuning of external dimension of our personality the final two stages leading to Samadhi (Self Realization) are impossible.

Thus a holistic approach is necessary.By following the eight limbs of yoga, individuals synchronize their mind, body, and soul. Each limb builds upon the others, creating a holistic approach to self-realization and inner harmony.

Through ethical conduct, physical postures, breath control, and meditation, practitioners can deepen their spiritual connection, quiet the mind, and experience profound states of awareness and bliss.

How is Samadhi reached?

It may be surprising to many of us but we all have been experiencing a state of Samadhi on a daily basis during dreamless deep sleep.

Our mind and senses are suspended in deep sleep and the only observer of that state is our true self. However, the absence of mind during this process inhibits us from recalling details of that state.

We have a vague feeling of having enjoyed that state after we wake up and as we all know, sleep is essential for our continued wellbeing.

So we connect with our true self on a regular basis. The fact of the matter is that our true conscious self is the ONLY observer of all our worldly experiences.

Our mind , senses and body are just plain inert matter being made to appear live by the power of the conscious self.

During Samadhi we attempt a voluntary reunion with this true self by process of meditation. Thus meditation is essential for realizing our true self.

Even in Bhakti (Devotion) yoga the ultimate union with Divine is considered to be a meditative surrender of our limited self to the Divine within.

Samadhi is actually a fourth state also called Turiya (numeral 4 in Sanskrit) in which we enter while fully awake by a process of stilling the perturbations in our mind. The other three are our waking, dream and deep sleep states.

Samadhi is deemed to have taken place when our mind is completely still, much like the placid water of a clean lake, reflecting the Moon from the night sky. The Moon is our true self.

There is no hard boundary separating the two phases viz. Sadhna and Samadhi. The eight limbs of Ashtanga Yoga consists of the first preparatory steps connected with ourselves and the environment we live in.

They are preparations to ensure that we progress smoothly through Dharna (Concentration) and Dhyan (Meditation). Effective meditation increases our possibility to get a glimpse of divinity within. **Figure 2** attempts to capture this process towards self-realization.

This process entails a very high proportion of actual practice. Like Cycling, Swimming or Dancing can not be learnt by watching YouTube videos alone and actual practice is necessary, same is the case with Yoga.

This spiritual journey of a seeker can be understood by a metaphor of an Aircraft getting airborne.

Preparatory Sadhna is akin to the ground crew working on it to ensure it's airworthiness. The process of taxiing to the runway takeoff point is like Dharna.

The takeoff run with full throttle is equivalent to Dhyan. Only when an aircraft reaches a critical speed can it get unstuck from the runway and get airborne. Similarly the Dhyan has to be firm to reach the Samadhi stage.

Once airborne aircraft gets over it's earlier limitations of not being able to travel across unpaved lands, rivers or mountains. Similarly a seeker in Samadhi stage transcends the earlier limitation of his mind and experiences a new found freedom or liberation.

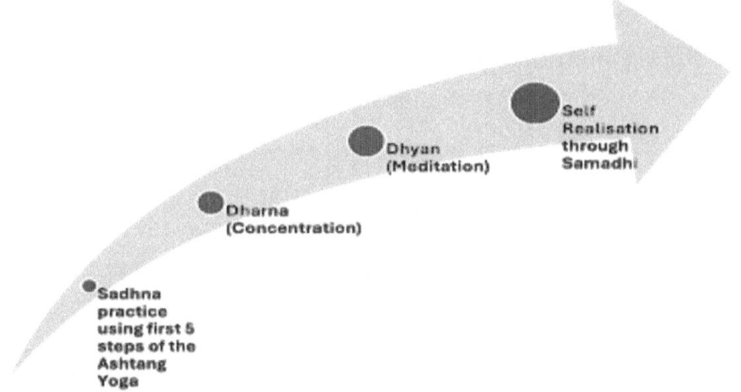

Figure 2: Process towards Self-Realisation

It is observed that a seeker may have apprehension in following the preparatory phase of observance of five Yamas, five Niyamas, stabilizing of Asan (Physical Exercises to strengthen the body), Pranayama (Breathing Exercises) and Pratyahara (Withdrawal of senses from world objects).

It is recommended that a seeker may motivate oneself to take the initial baby steps on this path, by appreciation of the immense value that the glimpse of the divine within provides them at the end of the long tunnel of spiritual Sadhna.

Another factor that inhibits us on this path is the fear of the unknown. The very idea of losing our existing concept of self to a very nebulous construct of divine self and consequences of this transformation on our 'business as usual' life, acts as a damper.

However, this fear is totally unfounded. A realized person is able to lead life with much better control on their interactions with the world around them.

Many insecurities and dissipation of our energies in useless pursuits give way to a more holistic approach to life and our relations with others including our immediate family and friends become better.

Having allayed these fears of the seeker, we may take a brief look at the actual process. Though this journey is a personal quest, the need of a teacher/guide (Guru) to guide is emphasized. Even for the Sadhna phase, the role of a suitable guide or a course of instruction is highly recommended.

Like in any discipline, the need to have our concepts clarified through self-study (Svadhyaya) and reflection (Manan) is essential to get the critical mass of detachment (Vairagya) from worldly indulgences.

Yoga Sutra, is one of the most detailed maps of higher consciousness; it deals primarily with the nature of mind, and with how the mind is transformed through different stages of samadhi (higher consciousness) until the liberated state, or kaivalya, finally appears.

Samadhi Pada is the opening chapter of Patanjali's Yog-Darshan or Yoga Sutras. It consists of 51 sutras that delve into the concept of enlightenment and the path to self-realization.

The term "samadhi" refers to a state of deep concentration, meditation, and absorption where the individual's consciousness merges with the object of focus. In this state, the sense of separation between the observer and the observed dissolves, leading to profound inner realization.

Purpose of Yoga According to Samadhi Pada:

Patanjali explains that the purpose of yoga is to quiet the fluctuations of the mind, known as "vrittis." These mental fluctuations are the source of restlessness, distractions, and suffering.

By practicing yoga, one aims to still these mental fluctuations and experience the true nature of the self beyond the conditioned mind.

Chitta-Vritti-Nirodha: Stilling the Mind:

• A central concept in Samadhi Pada is "chitta-vritti-nirodha," which refers to the stilling or calming of the mind-stuff (chitta).

• Through various yogic practices, the seeker learns to quiet the mind, allowing it to settle into a state of stillness and clarity.

Overcoming Obstacles:

• The chapter discusses obstacles and distractions that hinder the attainment of samadhi. These include desires, attachments, aversions, and other mental disturbances.

• Patanjali presents a path for overcoming these obstacles through the practice of "abstinences" (yamas) and "observances" (niyamas).

Types of Samadhi:

1. **Savikalpa Samadhi**:

   - In this state, the mind is concentrated and still, but the merger with the object of focus is not yet complete.

   - The practitioner experiences a deep meditative absorption, but there is still a subtle sense of duality.

2. **Nirvikalpa Samadhi**:

   - This is the highest state of samadhi.

   - The mind is fully absorbed and merged with the object of focus, leading to a complete dissolution of the sense of self.

- In Nirvikalpa Samadhi, the seeker experiences oneness and unity with the divine or the true self.

Importance of Samadhi:

• Samadhi is considered the crowning achievement of yogic practice. It represents the apex of the yogic journey, where the seeker transcends ordinary consciousness and enters a state of profound realization.

• Attaining samadhi is crucial for achieving liberation (moksha) and self-realization.

In summary, Samadhi Pada establishes the fundamental principles of yoga, emphasizing the quieting of the mind and the practice of samadhi as a means to realize the true self. It invites seekers to explore the depths of their consciousness and experience the ultimate union with existence.

12. Integration of Patanjali Yoga Sutra in Daily Life

Introduction

This chapter is an attempt to help readers adapt the concepts of Patanjali yoga sutra to modern context. Our social milieu has changed profoundly and appropriate approaches are called for to benefit from ancient wisdom.

Bridging Ancient Wisdom and Modern Living

The Yoga Sutras of Patanjali, composed over two millennia ago, remain one of the most profound and practical guides for human development ever written. While these 196 aphorisms were originally intended for dedicated spiritual practitioners, their timeless wisdom offers invaluable guidance for anyone seeking to live with greater awareness, purpose, and inner peace in our contemporary world.

Patanjali's systematic approach to yoga—meaning "union" or "integration"—provides a comprehensive framework for harmonizing our thoughts, emotions, actions, and relationships. Far from being merely philosophical concepts, these sutras offer concrete tools for navigating the complexities of modern life, from managing stress and relationships to finding meaning and maintaining ethical integrity in our personal and professional endeavors.

This chapter explores how to weave the essential teachings of the Yoga Sutras into the fabric of daily existence, transforming ordinary activities into opportunities for growth, self-awareness, and spiritual development.

By understanding and applying these principles, we can cultivate a life of greater clarity, compassion, and authentic fulfillment.

The Foundation: Understanding Yoga as a Way of Life

Before examining specific practices, it's essential to understand Patanjali's definition of yoga itself. In the second sutra, he states: "Yoga is the cessation of fluctuations of the mind" (Yogash chitta-vritti-nirodhah). This doesn't mean suppressing thoughts or emotions, but rather developing the capacity to observe them without being overwhelmed or controlled by them.

In practical terms, this foundational principle invites us to approach daily life with what we might call "conscious presence"—the ability to remain centered and aware regardless of external circumstances. Whether we're stuck in traffic, dealing with a difficult colleague, or facing personal challenges, the practice of yoga offers us tools to maintain inner equilibrium while responding skillfully to life's demands.

This shift from reactive to responsive living forms the cornerstone of integrating yogic principles into daily life. Instead of being at the mercy of our immediate impulses and emotional reactions, we develop the capacity to pause, breathe, and choose our responses consciously.

The Eight-Limbed Path: A Practical Framework for Daily Living

Patanjali's Ashtanga (eight-limbed) path provides a comprehensive roadmap for integrating yogic principles into every aspect of life. Rather than viewing these as sequential steps, we can understand them as interconnected dimensions of conscious living that support and reinforce one another.

The Yamas: Ethical Guidelines for Relationships

The first limb, the yamas, consists of five ethical restraints that guide our interactions with others and the world around us. These aren't rigid rules but intelligent guidelines that, when practiced consistently, create harmony in our relationships and communities.

Ahimsa (Non-violence) extends far beyond physical harm to encompass our thoughts, words, and actions. In daily life, this might mean choosing compassionate communication over harsh criticism, both with others and in our internal dialogue. It involves being mindful of how our consumption choices affect other beings and the environment, and cultivating gentleness in our approach to personal growth and self-improvement.

Practically, ahimsa invites us to notice when we're being violent toward ourselves through negative self-talk, excessive self-criticism, or pushing our bodies beyond healthy limits. It encourages us to extend the same kindness to ourselves that we would offer to a dear friend.

Satya (Truthfulness) involves more than simply not lying; it calls us to live authentically and speak our truth with wisdom and compassion. This means being honest about our feelings, needs, and boundaries while considering the impact of our words on others. In professional settings, satya might manifest as having the courage to voice ethical concerns or admitting when we don't know something rather than pretending otherwise.

Asteya (Non-stealing) encompasses not taking what isn't freely given, including others' time, energy, or credit for their work. In our consumer culture, asteya invites us to examine our relationship with material possessions and consider whether our desires stem from genuine need or unconscious craving. It also means being punctual, prepared, and fully present when others share their time with us.

Brahmacharya (Energy management) traditionally referred to celibacy, but in contemporary application, it's better understood as conscious use of our vital energy. This involves being mindful of how we direct our physical, emotional, and mental energy—whether through our relationships, work, entertainment choices, or spiritual practices. It's about finding balance and not dissipating our energy in ways that leave us depleted or scattered.

Aparigraha (Non-possessiveness) encourages us to hold material possessions and even relationships lightly, without clinging or attachment. This doesn't mean being indifferent, but rather appreciating what we have without being defined by it or constantly craving more. In practice, aparigraha helps us find contentment with what we have while remaining open to change and loss as natural parts of life.

The Niyamas: Personal Observances for Inner Development

The second limb, the niyamas, focuses on personal practices that cultivate inner growth and self-awareness.

Saucha (Cleanliness) involves both external and internal purification. Beyond maintaining physical hygiene and clean living spaces, saucha includes purifying our mental and emotional states through practices like meditation, spending time in nature, and consuming uplifting content. It might mean decluttering our homes, choosing nourishing foods, or limiting exposure to negative media.

Santosha (Contentment) is perhaps one of the most challenging yet rewarding practices in our achievement-oriented culture. Santosha doesn't mean complacency or lack of ambition, but rather finding peace and satisfaction in the present moment while working toward meaningful goals. It involves appreciating what we have rather than constantly focusing on what we lack.

Tapas (Disciplined practice) refers to the sustained effort required for growth and transformation. In daily life, tapas manifests as the commitment to maintain beneficial practices even when we don't feel like it—whether that's regular exercise, meditation, healthy eating, or keeping promises to ourselves and others. It's the inner fire that helps us overcome inertia and resistance to positive change.

Svadhyaya (Self-study) involves both studying sacred texts and engaging in honest self-reflection. This might include reading inspirational literature, journaling, or simply taking time to examine our thoughts, motivations, and patterns of behavior. In our information-rich age, svadhyaya also means being discerning about what we choose to study and ensuring that our learning contributes to wisdom rather than mere intellectual accumulation.

Ishvara pranidhana (Surrender to the divine) invites us to acknowledge something greater than our individual ego and to approach life with humility and trust. This doesn't require belief in a specific deity but rather recognition that we're part of something larger than ourselves—whether we call it nature, the universe, or the interconnected web of existence. Practically, this might mean letting go of the need to control outcomes and trusting in the unfolding of life's process.

Pranayama: The Breath as Gateway to Presence

The fourth limb of Patanjali's path, pranayama (breath regulation), offers one of the most accessible and powerful tools for integrating yogic awareness into daily life. Our breath serves as a bridge between body and mind, and conscious breathing practices can instantly shift our state of consciousness and help us respond to challenges with greater clarity and calm.

Simple breathing techniques can be seamlessly integrated into daily routines. The practice of conscious deep breathing for a few minutes upon waking helps set a peaceful tone for the day. During stressful moments at work, taking three conscious breaths can create space for a more thoughtful response. Before important conversations or meetings, a brief breathing practice can help center our energy and intention.

The beauty of pranayama is its availability—we're always breathing, so we always have access to this tool for cultivating presence and inner stability. Regular practice gradually develops what Patanjali calls "the capacity for concentration," making it easier to maintain awareness and equanimity throughout daily activities.

Pratyahara: Managing Sensory Input in a Stimulating World

In our hyper-connected, media-saturated environment, Patanjali's teaching on pratyahara (withdrawal of the senses) is particularly relevant. This doesn't mean shutting ourselves off from the world, but rather developing the ability to consciously choose what we allow into our awareness.

Practical pratyahara might involve creating regular periods of digital detox, choosing media consumption mindfully, or simply taking breaks from external stimulation to reconnect with our inner landscape. It could mean eating meals without distractions, taking walks without headphones, or spending time in natural settings where our senses can rest and restore.

By practicing pratyahara, we develop the capacity to remain centered and clear-minded even in stimulating or chaotic environments. We become less reactive to external circumstances and more able to maintain our inner equilibrium regardless of what's happening around us.

Dharana and Dhyana: Cultivating Focus and Awareness

The practices of dharana (concentration) and dhyana (meditation) are often thought of as formal sitting practices, but they can be integrated into daily activities in numerous ways. Any activity performed with sustained, focused attention becomes a form of dharana—whether it's washing dishes, listening to a friend, or completing a work project.

The key is bringing what Buddhists call "beginner's mind" to familiar activities, approaching them with fresh attention and presence. This transforms routine tasks into opportunities for cultivating awareness and finding meaning in ordinary moments.

Regular formal meditation practice supports this integration by developing our capacity for sustained attention and present-moment awareness. Even ten minutes of daily meditation can significantly impact our ability to remain centered and conscious throughout the day.

Practical Integration Strategies

Morning Practices: Setting Intention for the Day

Beginning each day with conscious intention creates a foundation for integrating yogic principles into daily life. This might involve a few minutes of meditation, reading an inspiring verse, or simply setting an intention for how you want to show up in the world that day.

A simple morning practice might include: conscious breathing while still in bed, expressing gratitude for the new day, setting an intention aligned with yogic principles, and perhaps reading a sutra or inspirational text. This doesn't need to be lengthy—even five to ten minutes can significantly impact the quality of awareness you bring to the day.

Mindful Transitions: Creating Sacred Pauses

Our days are filled with transitions—from home to work, from one task to another, from interaction to interaction. These moments offer perfect opportunities to reconnect with yogic awareness. A conscious breath between activities, a moment of gratitude before meals, or a brief pause to center yourself before entering your home can transform these transitions into moments of practice.

These "sacred pauses" help prevent the unconscious momentum that often carries us through days without real presence or awareness. They create space for conscious choice and help maintain connection to our deeper intentions and values.

Work as Spiritual Practice

Our professional lives offer rich opportunities for practicing yogic principles. Approaching work with the attitude of karma yoga—selfless service—can transform even mundane tasks into spiritual practice. This means focusing on the quality of our effort and attention rather than being attached to specific outcomes.

Practicing the yamas and niyamas in professional settings might involve speaking truthfully in meetings (satya), being punctual and prepared (asteya), managing our energy wisely throughout the workday (brahmacharya), and maintaining ethical standards even under pressure (ahimsa).

Relationships as Mirrors for Growth

Our relationships with family, friends, and colleagues provide constant opportunities to practice yogic principles. Every interaction offers a chance to practice compassion, truthfulness, and presence. Conflicts become opportunities to practice non-violence in our speech and thoughts, while daily interactions allow us to cultivate qualities like patience, understanding, and genuine listening.

Patanjali's teachings remind us that our reactions to others often reflect our own inner states and unresolved patterns. By bringing yogic awareness to our relationships, we can use them as mirrors for self-understanding and growth.

Overcoming Common Challenges

Dealing with Resistance and Inconsistency

One of the greatest challenges in integrating yogic principles into daily life is maintaining consistency, especially when old patterns feel more comfortable or convenient. Patanjali acknowledges this in his teachings about the obstacles to practice (antarayas) and offers practical guidance for working with resistance.

The key is starting small and building gradually. Rather than attempting to transform everything at once, choose one or two principles to focus on consistently. As these become more natural, you can gradually expand your practice to include other aspects of the yogic path.

Self-compassion is crucial during this process. Patanjali emphasizes that practice should be "steady and comfortable" (sthira sukham). This means finding a sustainable approach that honors your current circumstances and capacity while still encouraging growth.

Balancing Idealism with Practical Reality

The yogic path calls us toward high ideals, but it's important to approach these with wisdom and flexibility. Patanjali himself acknowledges that complete mastery of these principles is a lifelong journey, not a destination to be reached quickly.

The goal isn't perfection but rather gradual progress and increasing awareness. Each moment offers a fresh opportunity to choose a more conscious response, regardless of how we've acted in the past. This perspective helps maintain motivation while avoiding the discouragement that can come from setting unrealistic expectations.

Maintaining Practice During Difficult Times

Life inevitably brings challenges—illness, loss, relationship difficulties, financial stress, and other forms of suffering. These times test our commitment to yogic principles and often reveal how deeply our practice has taken root.

Patanjali's teachings suggest that difficulties are not obstacles to practice but rather opportunities to deepen our understanding and compassion. During challenging times, our practice might need to become simpler and more gentle, but it can also become more essential as a source of stability and wisdom.

The Fruits of Practice: Transformation Through Integration

As yogic principles become more integrated into daily life, practitioners often notice subtle but significant shifts in their experience. There's typically a growing sense of inner stability that isn't dependent on external circumstances, increased clarity in decision-making, and a natural expansion of compassion and understanding.

Relationships often improve as we become less reactive and more present with others. Work becomes more fulfilling as we approach it with greater consciousness and purpose. Even mundane activities can become sources of joy and meaning when approached with awareness and appreciation.

Perhaps most importantly, there's often a growing sense of alignment between our deepest values and our daily actions. This integrity creates a foundation for authentic happiness and fulfillment that doesn't depend on constantly changing external conditions.

Advanced Integration: Living the Sutras as a Complete Way of Life

As practice matures, the distinction between "yogic practice" and "daily life" begins to dissolve. Instead of compartmentalizing spiritual practice into specific times or activities, consciousness becomes a continuous thread running through all experiences.

This doesn't mean being serious or solemn all the time, but rather maintaining an underlying awareness and intentionality that infuses ordinary activities with meaning and purpose. Laughter, play, and joy become expressions of yogic awareness rather than distractions from it.

At this stage, practitioners often find that they naturally embody yogic principles without constantly thinking about them. Compassion, truthfulness, and presence become natural expressions of their being rather than effortful practices.

Conclusion: The Timeless Relevance of Ancient Wisdom

The Yoga Sutras of Patanjali offer a comprehensive and practical approach to human development that remains as relevant today as it was two thousand years ago. While the external conditions of life have changed dramatically, the fundamental challenges of being human—managing our thoughts and emotions, relating skillfully to others, finding meaning and purpose, and dealing with change and uncertainty—remain constant.

By integrating these timeless teachings into our contemporary lives, we can navigate modern challenges with greater wisdom, compassion, and inner stability. The sutras don't ask us to retreat from the world but rather to engage with it more consciously and skillfully.

The journey of integration is itself a practice of patience and persistence. Like a river gradually carving its path through rock, consistent application of yogic principles slowly but surely transforms the landscape of our lives. Each moment offers a new opportunity to choose awareness over unconsciousness, compassion over reaction, and wisdom over habit.

In this way, the ancient path of yoga becomes a thoroughly modern approach to living with integrity, purpose, and joy. The sutras remind us that transformation is possible at any moment and that the tools for creating a meaningful life are always available within us, waiting to be discovered and applied with dedication and love.

Through this integration, we not only transform our own lives but contribute to the healing and awakening of our communities and world. In embodying these principles, we become living examples of what's possible when ancient wisdom meets contemporary life, creating ripples of positive change that extend far beyond our individual experience.

The invitation of the Yoga Sutras is both simple and profound: to wake up to the fullness of life and to express our highest potential in every moment. This is not a destination to reach but a way of traveling, not a goal to achieve but a quality of presence to embody. In accepting this invitation, we discover that the path itself is the destination, and that every step taken with awareness is a step toward the ultimate goal of yoga—the integration of all aspects of our being into a harmonious and awakened whole.

I wish that the contents of this book set you on a journey that besides bestowing you with excellent health puts you in touch with your true self. May God bless you!

Appendix 'A'

Comprehensive Cellular Biology Glossary

A

Actin - A globular protein that forms microfilaments, crucial for cell structure, movement, and muscle contraction.

Active Transport - Energy-requiring process that moves substances across cell membranes against concentration gradients.

Adenosine Triphosphate (ATP) - The primary energy currency of cells, storing and releasing energy for cellular processes.

Aerobic Respiration - Cellular process that uses oxygen to break down glucose and produce ATP in mitochondria.

Allele - Alternative forms of a gene that occupy the same position on homologous chromosomes.

Amino Acid - Building blocks of proteins, containing amino and carboxyl groups.

Anaerobic Respiration - Cellular respiration that occurs without oxygen, producing less ATP than aerobic respiration.

Anaphase - Stage of mitosis where sister chromatids separate and move to opposite poles of the cell.

Antibody - Y-shaped proteins produced by B cells that bind to specific antigens.

Antigen - Foreign substance that triggers an immune response in the body.

Apoptosis - Programmed cell death, a controlled process of cellular suicide.

Archaea - Single-celled prokaryotic organisms distinct from bacteria, often found in extreme environments.

B

Bacteria - Single-celled prokaryotic organisms lacking a membrane-bound nucleus.

Base Pair - Two complementary nucleotides joined by hydrogen bonds in DNA (A-T, G-C).

Binary Fission - Asexual reproduction method used by prokaryotes where one cell divides into two identical cells.

Biomembrane - Selective barrier composed of phospholipids that surrounds cells and organelles.

Bivalent - Pair of homologous chromosomes joined together during meiosis.

C

Carbohydrate - Organic molecules composed of carbon, hydrogen, and oxygen, serving as energy sources and structural components.

Cell Cycle - Ordered sequence of events leading to cell division, including G1, S, G2, and M phases.

Cell Theory - Fundamental principle stating that all living things are made of cells, cells are the basic unit of life, and all cells come from pre-existing cells.

Cell Wall - Rigid protective layer surrounding plant cells, fungi, and bacteria.

Centromere - Constricted region of a chromosome where sister chromatids are joined.

Centrosome - Organelle containing two centrioles that organizes microtubules and helps in cell division.

Chaperone Protein - Proteins that assist in proper protein folding and prevent misfolding.

Chloroplast - Organelle in plant cells where photosynthesis occurs, containing chlorophyll.

Chromatin - Complex of DNA and proteins found in the nucleus of eukaryotic cells.

Chromosome - Structure containing DNA and proteins that carries genetic information.

Cilium - Short, hair-like projection from cells used for movement or moving substances.

Codon - Three-nucleotide sequence in mRNA that codes for a specific amino acid.

Complementary Base Pairing - Specific pairing of nucleotides (A with T/U, G with C) in DNA and RNA.

Crossing Over - Exchange of genetic material between homologous chromosomes during meiosis.

Cyclins - Proteins that regulate progression through the cell cycle.

Cytoplasm - Gel-like substance inside cells where organelles are suspended and many cellular processes occur.

Cytoskeleton - Network of protein filaments that provides structural support and shape to cells.

D

Differentiation - Process by which cells become specialized for specific functions.

Diffusion - Passive movement of substances from high to low concentration.

Diploid - Cells containing two complete sets of chromosomes (2n).

DNA (Deoxyribonucleic Acid) - Double-stranded nucleic acid that stores genetic information.

DNA Replication - Process of copying DNA before cell division.

Dominant - Allele that is expressed when present in heterozygous condition.

E

Electron Transport Chain - Series of protein complexes that transfer electrons and pump protons to generate ATP.

Endocytosis - Process by which cells take in materials by engulfing them with the cell membrane.

Endoplasmic Reticulum (ER) - Network of membranes in eukaryotic cells involved in protein and lipid synthesis.

Enzyme - Protein that catalyzes biochemical reactions by lowering activation energy.

Eukaryote - Organism whose cells have a membrane-bound nucleus and organelles.

Exocytosis - Process by which cells expel materials by fusing vesicles with the cell membrane.

Exon - Coding sequence in a gene that is expressed in the final mRNA.

F

Facilitated Diffusion - Passive transport of substances across membranes using transport proteins.

Fermentation - Anaerobic process that converts sugars to acids, gases, or alcohol.

Flagellum - Long, whip-like projection used for cell movement.

Fluid Mosaic Model - Model describing cell membranes as flexible structures with embedded proteins.

G

Gamete - Reproductive cell (sperm or egg) containing half the normal chromosome number.

Gene - Specific DNA sequence that codes for a particular trait or protein.

Gene Expression - Process by which genetic information is used to synthesize proteins.

Genetic Code - Set of rules by which DNA and RNA sequences are translated into proteins.

Genome - Complete set of genetic material in an organism.

Genotype - Genetic makeup of an organism.

Glucose - Simple sugar that serves as a primary energy source for cells.

Glycolysis - Metabolic pathway that breaks down glucose to produce ATP and pyruvate.

Golgi Apparatus - Organelle that modifies, packages, and ships proteins from the ER.

H

Haploid - Cells containing one complete set of chromosomes (n).

Heterozygous - Having two different alleles for a particular gene.

Histone - Proteins around which DNA winds to form nucleosomes.

Homeostasis - Maintenance of stable internal conditions in cells and organisms.

Homologous Chromosomes - Chromosome pairs with the same genes but possibly different alleles.

Homozygous - Having two identical alleles for a particular gene.

Hydrolysis - Chemical reaction that breaks bonds using water molecules.

I

Intermediate Filaments - Cytoskeletal components that provide structural stability to cells.

Interphase - Period of cell cycle between divisions when cells grow and replicate DNA.

Intron - Non-coding sequence in a gene that is removed during RNA processing.

Ion Channel - Protein that allows specific ions to pass through cell membranes.

Isotonic - Solution with equal solute concentration on both sides of a membrane.

K

Karyotype - Visual representation of an organism's complete set of chromosomes.

Kinase - Enzyme that adds phosphate groups to other molecules.

Krebs Cycle - Series of reactions in mitochondria that produces energy carriers from acetyl-CoA.

L

Lipid - Hydrophobic biological molecules including fats, oils, and membrane components.

Lysosome - Organelle containing digestive enzymes that break down waste materials.

M

Meiosis - Type of cell division that produces gametes with half the chromosome number.

Membrane Potential - Electrical charge difference across a cell membrane.

Messenger RNA (mRNA) - RNA molecule that carries genetic information from DNA to ribosomes.

Metaphase - Stage of cell division when chromosomes align at the cell's equator.

Microfilament - Thinnest component of the cytoskeleton, made of actin.

Microtubule - Largest cytoskeletal component involved in cell shape and organelle movement.

Mitochondrion - Organelle responsible for cellular respiration and ATP production.

Mitosis - Type of cell division that produces two identical diploid cells.

Mutation - Change in DNA sequence that may affect gene function.

N

Nucleic Acid - Large molecules (DNA and RNA) that store and transmit genetic information.

Nucleoid - Region in prokaryotic cells where genetic material is located.

Nucleolus - Dense region within the nucleus where ribosomal RNA is synthesized.

Nucleosome - DNA wrapped around histone proteins, forming the basic unit of chromatin.

Nucleotide - Building block of nucleic acids, consisting of a base, sugar, and phosphate.

Nucleus - Membrane-bound organelle containing the cell's genetic material.

O

Oncogene - Gene that, when mutated or overexpressed, can contribute to cancer development.

Organelle - Specialized structure within cells that performs specific functions.

Osmosis - Diffusion of water across a selectively permeable membrane.

Oxidative Phosphorylation - Process that produces ATP using energy from electron transport chain.

P

Passive Transport - Movement of substances across membranes without energy input.

Peptide Bond - Chemical bond linking amino acids in proteins.

Peroxisome - Organelle involved in lipid metabolism and detoxification.

Phenotype - Observable characteristics of an organism resulting from genetic and environmental factors.

Phospholipid - Major component of cell membranes with hydrophilic head and hydrophobic tails.

Photosynthesis - Process by which plants convert light energy into chemical energy.

Plasmid - Small, circular DNA molecule found in bacteria, separate from chromosomal DNA.

Prokaryote - Organism lacking a membrane-bound nucleus and organelles.

Prophase - First stage of mitosis when chromosomes condense and become visible.

Protein - Large molecules composed of amino acids that perform various cellular functions.

Protein Synthesis - Process of making proteins from amino acids using genetic instructions.

R

Recessive - Allele that is only expressed when present in homozygous condition.

Ribonucleic Acid (RNA) - Single-stranded nucleic acid involved in protein synthesis and gene regulation.

Ribosome - Cellular structure where protein synthesis occurs.

RNA Polymerase - Enzyme that synthesizes RNA from DNA template.

S

Signal Transduction - Process by which cells detect, process, and respond to external signals.

Spindle Fibers - Protein structures that move chromosomes during cell division.

Stem Cell - Undifferentiated cell capable of developing into various cell types.

Substrate - Molecule upon which an enzyme acts.

T

Telomere - Protective DNA-protein structures at chromosome ends.

Transcription - Process of synthesizing RNA from DNA template.

Transfer RNA (tRNA) - RNA molecule that brings amino acids to ribosomes during protein synthesis.

Translation - Process of synthesizing proteins from mRNA instructions.

Tumor Suppressor Gene - Gene that prevents uncontrolled cell growth when functioning normally.

V

Vacuole - Large storage compartment in plant cells.

Vesicle - Small membrane-bound sac that transports materials within cells.

Virus - Infectious agent that requires host cells to reproduce.

Z

Zygote - Diploid cell formed by fusion of male and female gametes.

This glossary covers fundamental terms in cellular biology. Each term represents a key concept essential for understanding how cells function, reproduce, and interact with their environment.

Appendix 'B'

Comprehensive Meditation Practice Glossary

A

Anapanasati - Mindfulness of breathing; a fundamental Buddhist meditation practice focusing on breath awareness.

Anchor - Primary object of attention in meditation (breath, mantra, visualization) that serves as a reference point.

Awareness - Pure consciousness or knowing quality of mind that observes without judgment.

Attention - Focused mental energy directed toward a specific object or experience.

Absorption - Deep state of concentration where the meditator becomes fully immersed in the meditation object.

Altered State - Non-ordinary state of consciousness that may arise during deep meditation.

Alertness - Quality of wakeful attention maintained during meditation practice.

Acceptance - Non-resistant attitude toward whatever arises in meditation experience.

Arising - The moment when thoughts, sensations, or emotions first appear in awareness.

Attachment - Mental clinging or identification with thoughts, emotions, or experiences.

B

Body Scan - Systematic meditation technique involving conscious attention to different parts of the body.

Breath Counting - Meditation practice of counting breaths to develop concentration.

Buddha Nature - Inherent potential for awakening present in all beings.

Beginner's Mind - Attitude of openness and curiosity, free from preconceptions.

Bell - Sound used to begin or end meditation sessions, or as meditation object.

Bliss - State of profound happiness or joy that may arise in deep meditation.

Being Mode - State of simply existing in present awareness without doing or achieving.

Bare Attention - Pure noticing without analysis, judgment, or mental commentary.

Breathing Space - Brief mindfulness practice creating pause between activities.

Boundless - Experience of consciousness without perceived limits or boundaries.

C

Concentration - Sustained, focused attention on a single object or experience.

Contemplation - Reflective meditation involving sustained inquiry into specific themes.

Cushion - Traditional meditation seat, typically round zafu or rectangular zabuton.

Centering - Process of gathering scattered attention into unified focus.

Clarity - Quality of clear, undisturbed awareness free from mental fog.

Calm Abiding - Shamatha in Sanskrit; meditation developing mental stability and peace.

Compassion - Loving response to suffering in oneself and others.

Choiceless Awareness - Open monitoring meditation without selecting specific objects.

Cycling - Natural rhythm of attention moving between focus and distraction.

Cushion Time - Duration spent in formal seated meditation practice.

D

Dharana - Sanskrit term for concentration; sustained attention on single object.

Dhyana - Sanskrit term for meditation; sustained flow of awareness.

Distraction - Mental movement away from chosen meditation object.

Dullness - Mental state characterized by lack of clarity or energy.

Deep Listening - Meditative practice of attentive, non-judgmental hearing.

Dropping - Letting go of thoughts, emotions, or sensations without resistance.

Direct Experience - Immediate, non-conceptual knowing through present-moment awareness.

Dissolution - Experience of boundaries between self and environment fading.

Daily Practice - Regular meditation routine integrated into everyday life.

Devotional Meditation - Practice involving love, surrender, or connection with sacred.

E

Emptiness - Buddhist concept of lack of inherent, independent existence.

Equanimity - Balanced state of mind remaining stable through changing experiences.

Effortless - Natural state of meditation without forcing or striving.

Energy - Subtle life force or vitality experienced during meditation.

Enlightenment - State of complete awakening or liberation from suffering.

Embodied - Grounded awareness including bodily sensations and presence.

Expansion - Experience of consciousness extending beyond normal boundaries.

Emotional Regulation - Capacity to maintain balance with difficult emotions.

Entering - Process of settling into meditative state from ordinary consciousness.

Exhale - Out-breath phase often emphasized in breathing meditation.

F

Focus - Concentrated attention directed toward specific meditation object.

Flow State - Effortless absorption where self-consciousness disappears.

Formal Practice - Structured meditation sessions with designated time and place.

Flexibility - Mental quality allowing adaptation to changing meditation experiences.

Friendliness - Gentle, kind attitude toward oneself during practice.

Falling Away - Natural dropping of thoughts, tensions, or mental constructs.

Field of Awareness - Spacious quality of consciousness containing all experience.

Feeling Tone - Pleasant, unpleasant, or neutral quality of each experience.

Full Catastrophe Living - Mindful engagement with life's complete range of experiences.

Formless - Meditation practices without specific visualization or conceptual object.

G

Guided Meditation - Practice led by teacher's verbal instructions.

Gong - Sound instrument used to mark meditation periods or as focus object.

Grounding - Establishing stable connection with earth, body, or present moment.

Glimpse - Brief moment of expanded awareness or insight.

Gentle Persistence - Sustained practice with kind, non-forcing attitude.

Gap - Space between thoughts where pure awareness can be recognized.

Guru - Spiritual teacher providing meditation instruction and guidance.

Grace - Effortless arising of meditative states or spiritual experiences.

Group Practice - Meditation done together with others in community setting.

Gratitude Practice - Meditation cultivating appreciation and thankfulness.

H

Hara - Energy center below navel; focus point in some meditation traditions.

Heart Center - Chest area emphasized in loving-kindness and compassion practices.

Hindrances - Mental obstacles to meditation: desire, aversion, restlessness, dullness, doubt.

Here and Now - Present moment awareness; fundamental focus of mindfulness.

Holding - Gentle attention that neither grasps nor pushes away experience.

Higher Self - Transcendent aspect of identity accessed through deep meditation.

Healing - Therapeutic benefits arising from regular meditation practice.

Harmony - Balanced state where all aspects of experience feel integrated.

Humming - Sound meditation using vocal vibrations for focus and calming.

Habit Formation - Process of establishing consistent meditation routine.

I

Insight - Direct understanding or wisdom arising from meditation practice.

Informal Practice - Mindfulness applied to daily activities and routine tasks.

Inner Silence - Quiet mental space free from mental commentary.

Intention - Purpose or motivation underlying meditation practice.

Inquiry - Investigative approach exploring the nature of experience.

Impermanence - Understanding that all phenomena are constantly changing.

Integration - Process of incorporating meditation insights into daily life.

Interconnectedness - Recognition of fundamental unity underlying apparent separation.

Inner Observer - Witnessing aspect of consciousness that watches all experience.

Inhale - In-breath phase often emphasized in breathing meditation.

J

Jhana - Deep absorption states described in Buddhist meditation literature.

Just Sitting - Shikantaza in Zen; open awareness meditation without specific object.

Journey - Understanding meditation practice as ongoing path of development.

Joy - Natural happiness arising from peaceful, concentrated states.

Judgment - Mental evaluation that meditation practice learns to observe and release.

Japa - Repetitive recitation of mantra or sacred phrase.

Jewel - Precious insight or realization discovered through practice.

Joining - Merging attention completely with meditation object.

Jump - Sudden shift in consciousness or awareness during practice.

Juice - Vitality or energy experienced during or after meditation.

K

Koan - Zen meditation using paradoxical questions to transcend logical thinking.

Kindness - Gentle, friendly attitude cultivated toward self and others.

Kinhin - Walking meditation practiced in Zen tradition.

Knowing - Pure awareness or consciousness that recognizes all experience.

Kundalini - Spiritual energy that may awaken through intensive meditation practice.

Karma - Law of cause and effect; understanding how actions create consequences.

Kernel - Essential seed or core insight arising from meditation.

Key - Particular technique or understanding that unlocks deeper practice.

Kensho - Zen term for initial glimpse of enlightened awareness.

Kriya - Purification technique using breath, movement, or visualization.

L

Loving-Kindness - Metta meditation cultivating unconditional love and goodwill.

Letting Go - Release of attachment to thoughts, emotions, or experiences.

Labeling - Mental noting technique identifying types of arising experience.

Luminosity - Clear, bright quality of pure awareness.

Lineage - Traditional chain of teaching transmission from teacher to student.

Lotus Position - Classic cross-legged sitting posture for meditation.

Light - Inner radiance or illumination experienced in deep states.

Longing - Deep desire for truth, peace, or spiritual fulfillment.

Listening - Receptive attention to sounds, silence, or inner guidance.

Liberation - Freedom from mental suffering and limitation.

M

Mindfulness - Present-moment awareness with acceptance and non-judgment.

Mantra - Sacred word, phrase, or sound repeated for concentration and transformation.

Metta - Loving-kindness; cultivation of unconditional love and goodwill.

Meditation Object - Specific focus chosen for concentration practice.

Monkey Mind - Restless, scattered mental state jumping between thoughts.

Movement Meditation - Practice incorporating gentle physical movement.

Mudra - Hand position or gesture supporting meditation practice.

Moment - Brief unit of experience; present-moment awareness.

Mental Noting - Technique of briefly labeling arising thoughts and sensations.

Momentum - Building energy and continuity in meditation practice.

N

Non-Dual - Recognition that observer and observed are not separate.

No-Mind - State of consciousness without conceptual thinking.

Noting - Mental labeling technique for observing arising experiences.

Now - Present moment; the only time when life actually occurs.

Non-Attachment - Freedom from clinging while remaining fully engaged.

Natural State - Effortless condition of pure awareness without modification.

Nimitta - Sign or mental image arising in concentrated meditation states.

Noble Silence - Periods of not speaking to support contemplative practice.

Nirvana - Ultimate peace; cessation of suffering through complete awakening.

Nurturing - Caring, supportive attitude toward developing meditation practice.

O

Open Awareness - Spacious meditation monitoring whatever arises without choosing objects.

One-Pointedness - Complete unification of attention on single meditation object.

Observer - Witnessing aspect of consciousness that watches all mental activity.

Om - Sacred sound often used as mantra for concentration and devotion.

Openness - Receptive quality of mind willing to experience whatever arises.

Ordinary Mind - Natural state of awareness before mental elaboration.

Obstacles - Challenges or hindrances encountered in meditation practice.

Oceanic - Boundless, flowing quality of expanded conscious states.

Offering - Devotional attitude of giving practice for benefit of all beings.

Oneness - Direct experience of fundamental unity underlying apparent diversity.

P

Present Moment - Immediate experience happening right now.

Posture - Physical position maintained during formal meditation practice.

Pranayama - Breath control practices supporting meditation and energy cultivation.

Purification - Cleansing process releasing mental and emotional impurities.

Presence - Quality of being fully here and available to immediate experience.

Peace - Fundamental tranquility underlying all mental states and activities.

Pointing Out - Direct introduction to nature of mind by qualified teacher.

Pure Land - Devotional practice visualizing enlightened realm of peace.

Plateau - Period in practice where progress seems to level off.

Psychic - Subtle perceptions or abilities that may develop through practice.

Q

Quieting - Natural settling of mental activity in meditation.

Quality - Particular characteristic or flavor of meditative experience.

Questioning - Inquiry practice investigating nature of self and reality.

Quiescence - Deep tranquility and mental stillness.

Quest - Spiritual search or journey toward understanding and awakening.

Quickening - Acceleration of spiritual development through intensive practice.

Quintessence - Pure essence or most refined aspect of meditative realization.

Quantum - Sudden leap or breakthrough in understanding or experience.

Quelling - Pacifying agitated mental states through skillful practice.

Quote - Inspiring teaching or instruction supporting meditation practice.

R

Refuge - Source of protection and guidance on spiritual path.

Retreat - Extended period of intensive meditation practice.

Relaxation - Natural ease and softness arising from letting go of tension.

Recognition - Direct knowing of awareness itself as fundamental nature.

Ripening - Gradual maturation of meditation insights and realizations.

Refuge Tree - Visualization practice connecting with lineage of teachers and wisdom.

Resting - Natural settling into stillness without effort or manipulation.

Reverence - Respectful appreciation for teachings, teachers, and sacred dimension.

Rhythm - Natural flow or pattern in breathing, walking, or chanting practices.

Radiance - Luminous quality of pure awareness when mental obscurations clear.

S

Samadhi - Deep absorption or unity consciousness in meditation.

Shamatha - Calm abiding; developing mental stability and peace.

Sati - Pali term for mindfulness; clear awareness of present experience.

Satsang - Gathering with others for spiritual practice and discussion.

Silence - Absence of mental commentary; inner quietude.

Stillness - Quality of non-movement in body and mind.

Surrender - Letting go of personal will and control to deeper wisdom.

Stream Entry - First stage of awakening in Buddhist meditation path.

Spaciousness - Open, unlimited quality of pure awareness.

Subtle - Refined levels of experience accessible through deep meditation.

T

Transcendence - Going beyond ordinary limitations of self and experience.

Tranquility - Deep peace and mental calm developed through meditation.

Third Eye - Energy center between eyebrows associated with inner vision.

Tonglen - Tibetan practice of breathing in suffering and breathing out relief.

Teacher - Guide providing instruction and support for meditation practice.

Transformation - Fundamental change in understanding and experience through practice.

Tradition - Lineage of teachings and practices passed down through generations.

Technique - Specific method or approach used in meditation practice.

Timelessness - Experience of being beyond past and future in eternal now.

Trust - Confidence in practice, teachings, and natural unfolding of awareness.

U

Unity - Direct experience of fundamental oneness underlying apparent diversity.

Unification - Integration of scattered attention into coherent, focused awareness.

Unconditional - Love, acceptance, or awareness not dependent on circumstances.

Understanding - Wisdom arising from direct meditation experience.

Unwinding - Natural release of physical and mental tensions.

Upstream - Moving attention back to its source in pure awareness.

Ultimate - Absolute level of truth beyond conventional, relative experience.

Unborn - Timeless, uncreated nature of pure consciousness.

Unknowing - Letting go of conceptual knowledge to access direct experience.

Union - Integration of different aspects of self or merger with meditation object.

V

Vipassana - Insight meditation investigating nature of experience and reality.

Visualization - Mental imagery practices using specific forms, colors, or scenes.

Vows - Commitments supporting ethical conduct and spiritual development.

Void - Empty, open space of pure awareness beyond mental content.

Virtue - Ethical conduct supporting and arising from meditation practice.

Vigilance - Alert awareness maintaining clear attention during practice.

Voice - Inner guidance or wisdom accessed through quiet contemplation.

Vastness - Unlimited, boundless quality of expanded conscious states.

Vibration - Subtle energy or frequency experienced in deep meditation.

Veil - Mental obscurations covering natural clarity of awareness.

W

Walking Meditation - Mindful movement practice using steps as meditation object.

Witness - Pure awareness that observes all mental and physical phenomena.

Wisdom - Understanding arising from direct experience rather than conceptual knowledge.

Wakefulness - Alert, clear quality of mind maintained during meditation.

Wholeness - Experience of complete integration and unified awareness.

Wonder - Natural awe and curiosity arising from expanded perception.

Warmth - Loving, compassionate quality accompanying deep meditation states.

Way - Path or method leading toward spiritual understanding and freedom.

Wordless - Direct experience beyond concepts and mental descriptions.

Willingness - Open attitude of receptivity to whatever arises in practice.

Y

Yoga - Union of individual and universal consciousness through practice.

Yielding - Soft surrender allowing natural unfolding of meditative experience.

Yearning - Deep longing for truth, peace, or spiritual fulfillment.

Yin - Receptive, passive quality emphasized in certain meditation approaches.

Yogi - Practitioner dedicated to spiritual development through meditation.

Yes - Accepting attitude embracing all aspects of meditation experience.

Yesterday Mind - Past-oriented thinking that meditation practice learns to release.

Yawning - Natural release that may occur as body relaxes in meditation.

Yielding - Allowing meditation to unfold naturally without force or control.

Youth - Fresh, beginner's mind approach regardless of age or experience.

Z

Zazen - "Just sitting" meditation practiced in Zen tradition.

Zen - Direct pointing to enlightened mind beyond words and concepts.

Zeal - Enthusiastic energy supporting dedicated meditation practice.

Zone - State of effortless flow and optimal performance.

Zendo - Meditation hall used for formal Zen practice.

Zero Point - Still center of pure awareness from which all experience arises.

Zephyr - Gentle, subtle movement of energy or breath during practice.

Zenith - Peak experience or highest attainment in meditation development.

Zest - Joyful energy and enthusiasm arising from spiritual practice.

Zigzag - Non-linear nature of spiritual development with its ups and downs.

This comprehensive glossary encompasses meditation terminology from Buddhist, Hindu, Zen, mindfulness, and contemporary approaches. These terms provide a complete vocabulary for understanding and discussing meditation practice, theory, and experience across different traditions and methodologies.

Bibliography

PART I: FOUNDATIONS

Chapter 1 - Consciousness and the Cosmos

1. Chalmers, D. J. (1996). The Conscious Mind: In Search of a Fundamental Theory. Oxford University Press.
2. Dehaene, S. (2014). Consciousness and the Brain: Deciphering How the Brain Codes Our Thoughts. Viking.
3. Deutsch, E. (1969). Advaita Vedanta: A Philosophical Reconstruction. University of Hawaii Press.
4. Hameroff, S., & Penrose, R. (2014). Consciousness in the universe: A review of the 'Orch OR' theory. Physics of Life Reviews, 11(1), 39-78.
5. James, W. (1902). The Varieties of Religious Experience: A Study in Human Nature. Longmans, Green & Co.
6. Koch, C. (2012). Consciousness: Confessions of a Romantic Reductionist. MIT Press. 7. Maharaj, N. (1973). I Am That: Talks with Sri Nisargadatta Maharaj. Acorn Press.
8. Nagel, T. (1974). What Is It Like to Be a Bat? The Philosophical Review, 83(4), 435-450.
9. Olivelle, P. (1998). The Early Upanishads: Annotated Text and Translation. Oxford University Press.
10. Penrose, R. (1989). The Emperor's New Mind: Concerning Computers, Minds, and the Laws of Physics. Oxford University Press.
11. Revonsuo, A. (2009). Consciousness: The Science of Subjectivity. Psychology Press.
12. Searle, J. R. (1997). The Mystery of Consciousness. New York Review of Books.
13. Shear, J. (ed.) (1997). Explaining Consciousness: The Hard Problem. MIT Press.

14. Stapp, H. P. (2007). Mindful Universe: Quantum Mechanics and the Participating Observer. Springer.
15. Thompson, E. (2014). Waking, Dreaming, Being: Self and Consciousness in Neuroscience, Meditation, and Philosophy. Columbia University Press.
16. Tononi, G. (2012). Integrated information theory of consciousness: an updated account. Archives Italiennes de Biologie, 150(2-3), 56-90.
17. Velmans, M. (2009). Understanding Consciousness. Routledge.
18. Wallace, B. A. (2007). Contemplative Science: Where Buddhism and Neuroscience Converge. Columbia University Press.
19. Wilber, K. (1997). The Eye of Spirit: An Integral Vision for a World Gone Slightly Mad. Shambhala.
20. Zeman, A. (2002). Consciousness: A User's Guide. Yale University Press.

Chapter 2: The Science of Self-Healing

1. Dispenza, J. (2014). You Are the Placebo: Making Your Mind Matter. Hay House, Inc.
2. Blackburn, E., & Epel, E. (2017). The Telomere Effect: A Revolutionary Approach to Living Younger, Healthier, Longer. Grand Central Publishing.
3. Kaptchuk, T. J., & Miller, F. G. (2015). Placebo effects in medicine. New England Journal of Medicine, 373(1), 8-9.
4. Wager, T. D., & Atlas, L. Y. (2015). The neuroscience of placebo effects: connecting context, learning and health. Nature Reviews Neuroscience, 16(7), 403-418.
5. Benedetti, F. (2014). Placebo Effects: Understanding the Mechanisms in Health and Disease. Oxford University Press.

6. Pert, C. B. (1997). Molecules of Emotion: Why You Feel the Way You Feel. Scribner.

Chapter 3: Understanding Your Inner Biology

1. Blackburn, E. H., Epel, E. S., & Lin, J. (2015). Human telomere biology: A contributory and interactive factor in aging, disease risks, and protection. Science, 350(6265), 1193-1198.
2. Epel, E. S. (2009). Telomeres in a life-span perspective: A new "psychobiomarker"? Current Directions in Psychological Science, 18(1), 6-10.
3. Schutte, N. S., & Malouff, J. M. (2014). A meta-analytic review of the effects of mindfulness meditation on telomerase activity. Psychoneuroendocrinology, 42, 45-48.
4. Ornish, D., Lin, J., Chan, J. M., Epel, E., Kemp, C., Weidner, G., ... & Blackburn, E. H. (2013). Effect of comprehensive lifestyle changes on telomerase activity and telomere length in men with biopsy-proven low-risk prostate cancer: 5-year follow-up of a descriptive pilot study. The Lancet Oncology, 14(11), 1112-1120.
5. Epel, E. S., Blackburn, E. H., Lin, J., Dhabhar, F. S., Adler, N. E., Morrow, J. D., & Cawthon, R. M. (2004). Accelerated telomere shortening in response to life stress. Proceedings of the National Academy of Sciences, 101(49), 17312-17315.

Chapter 4: The Power of Meditation

1. Goleman, D., & Davidson, R. J. (2017). Altered Traits: Science Reveals How Meditation Changes Your Mind, Brain, and Body. Avery.
2. Kabat-Zinn, J. (2013). Full Catastrophe Living: Using the Wisdom of Your Body and Mind to Face Stress, Pain, and Illness. Bantam Books.

3. Lazar, S. W., Kerr, C. E., Wasserman, R. H., Gray, J. R., Greve, D. N., Treadway, M. T., ... & Fischl, B. (2005). Meditation experience is associated with increased cortical thickness. Neuroreport, 16(17), 1893-1897.

4. Tang, Y. Y., Hölzel, B. K., & Posner, M. I. (2015). The neuroscience of mindfulness meditation. Nature Reviews Neuroscience, 16(4), 213-225.

5. Lutz, A., Slagter, H. A., Dunne, J. D., & Davidson, R. J. (2008). Attention regulation and monitoring in meditation. Trends in Cognitive Sciences, 12(4), 163-169.

PART II: THE MIND AS MEDICINE

Chapter 5: Breaking the Addiction to the Past

1. Dispenza, J. (2012). Breaking the Habit of Being Yourself: How to Lose Your Mind and Create a New One. Hay House, Inc.

2. Lipton, B. H. (2005). The Biology of Belief: Unleashing the Power of Consciousness, Matter and Miracles. Hay House, Inc.

3. Hanson, R. (2013). Hardwiring Happiness: The New Brain Science of Contentment, Calm, and Confidence. Harmony.

4. Hölzel, B. K., Lazar, S. W., Gard, T., Schuman-Olivier, Z., Vago, D. R., & Ott, U. (2011). How does mindfulness meditation work? Proposing mechanisms of action from a conceptual and neural perspective. Perspectives on Psychological Science, 6(6), 537-559.

5. Colloca, L., & Miller, F. G. (2011). The nocebo effect and its relevance for clinical practice. Psychosomatic Medicine, 73(7), 598-603.

Chapter 6: Cultivating Positive Expectancy

1. Siegel, D. J. (2010). Mindsight: The New Science of Personal Transformation. Bantam Books.
2. Seligman, M. E. (2012). Flourish: A Visionary New Understanding of Happiness and Well-being. Simon and Schuster.
3. Kirsch, I. (2010). The Emperor's New Drugs: Exploding the Antidepressant Myth. Basic Books.
4. Beauregard, M. (2012). Brain Wars: The Scientific Battle Over the Existence of the Mind and the Proof That Will Change the Way We Live Our Lives. HarperOne.
5. Watkins, T. D., Horan, J. J., & Rapee, R. M. (2012). Meta-analysis of imagery-guided treatment in clinical psychology. Journal of Cognitive Psychotherapy, 26(1), 50-64.

Chapter 7: Stress, Telomeres, and the Meditative Solution

1. Epel, E. S., Puterman, E., Lin, J., Blackburn, E., Lazaro, A., & Mendes, W. B. (2013). Wandering minds and aging cells. Clinical Psychological Science, 1(1), 75-83.
2. Sapolsky, R. M. (2004). Why Zebras Don't Get Ulcers. Henry Holt and Company.
3. Creswell, J. D., Pacilio, L. E., Lindsay, E. K., & Brown, K. W. (2014). Brief mindfulness meditation training alters psychological and neuroendocrine responses to social evaluative stress. Psychoneuroendocrinology, 44, 1-12.
4. Jacobs, T. L., Epel, E. S., Lin, J., Blackburn, E. H., Wolkowitz, O. M., Bridwell, D. A., ... & Saron, C. D. (2011). Intensive meditation training, immune cell telomerase activity, and psychological mediators. Psychoneuroendocrinology, 36(5), 664-681.

5. Dusek, J. A., Otu, H. H., Wohlhueter, A. L., Bhasin, M., Zerbini, L. F., Joseph, M. G., ... & Libermann, T. A. (2008). Genomic counter-stress changes induced by the relaxation response. PloS One, 3(7), e2576.

PART III: THE PRACTICE

Chapter 8: Meditation for Genetic Expression

1. Church, D. (2018). Mind to Matter: The Astonishing Science of How Your Brain Creates Material Reality. Hay House, Inc.
2. Rossi, E. L. (2002). The Psychobiology of Gene Expression: Neuroscience and Neurogenesis in Hypnosis and the Healing Arts. W. W. Norton & Company.
3. Bhasin, M. K., Dusek, J. A., Chang, B. H., Joseph, M. G., Denninger, J. W., Fricchione, G. L., ... & Libermann, T. A. (2013). Relaxation response induces temporal transcriptome changes in energy metabolism, insulin secretion and inflammatory pathways. PloS One, 8(5), e62817.
4. Kaliman, P., Álvarez-López, M. J., Cosín-Tomás, M., Rosenkranz, M. A., Lutz, A., & Davidson, R. J. (2014). Rapid changes in histone deacetylases and inflammatory gene expression in expert meditators. Psychoneuroendocrinology, 40, 96-107.
5. Lin, J., Epel, E., Cheon, J., Kroenke, C., Sinclair, E., Bigos, M., ... & Blackburn, E. (2010). Analyses and comparisons of telomerase activity and telomere length in human T and B cells: insights for epidemiology of telomere maintenance. Journal of Immunological Methods, 352(1-2), 71-80.

Chapter 9: The Emotional Connection

1. Davidson, R. J., & Begley, S. (2012). The Emotional Life of Your Brain: How Its Unique Patterns Affect the Way You Think, Feel, and Live—and How You Can Change Them. Hudson Street Press.

2. McCraty, R., & Zayas, M. A. (2014). Cardiac coherence, self-regulation, autonomic stability, and psychosocial well-being. Frontiers in Psychology, 5, 1090.

3. Fredrickson, B. L., Grewen, K. M., Coffey, K. A., Algoe, S. B., Firestine, A. M., Arevalo, J. M., ... & Cole, S. W. (2013). A functional genomic perspective on human well-being. Proceedings of the National Academy of Sciences, 110(33), 13684-13689.

4. O'Donovan, A., Lin, J., Dhabhar, F. S., Wolkowitz, O., Tillie, J. M., Blackburn, E., & Epel, E. (2009). Pessimism correlates with leukocyte telomere shortness and elevated interleukin-6 in post-menopausal women. Brain, Behavior, and Immunity, 23(4), 446-449.

5. Neff, K. D., & Germer, C. K. (2013). A pilot study and randomized controlled trial of the mindful self-compassion program. Journal of Clinical Psychology, 69(1), 28-44.

Chapter 10: Living in the Quantum Field

1. Dispenza, J. (2017). Becoming Supernatural: How Common People Are Doing the Uncommon. Hay House, Inc.

2. Radin, D. (2018). Real Magic: Ancient Wisdom, Modern Science, and a Guide to the Secret Power of the Universe. Harmony.

3. Schwartz, G. E., & Simon, W. L. (2007). The Energy Healing Experiments: Science Reveals Our Natural Power to Heal. Atria Books.

4. Oschman, J. L. (2015). Energy Medicine: The Scientific Basis. Elsevier Health Sciences.

5. McTaggart, L. (2008). The Field: The Quest for the Secret Force of the Universe. HarperCollins.

PART IV: PHILOSOPHY OF MEDITATION

Chapter 11: Patanjali Yoga Sutra

Ancient Texts:

1. Patanjali. Yoga Sutras (c. 1st-2nd century CE). Original Sanskrit text with 195-196 aphorisms on the theory and practice of yoga.
2. Vyasa. Yoga-Bhashya (Commentary on the Yoga Sutras, c. 4th-5th century CE). The earliest and most authoritative commentary on Patanjali's Yoga Sutras.
3. Vacaspati Misra. Tattva-Vaisharadi (c. 9th century CE). A sub-commentary on Vyasa's Yoga-Bhashya.
4. Vijnana Bhiksu. Yoga-Varttika (c. 16th century CE). Important traditional commentary reconciling Yoga with Vedanta philosophy.

Academic and Scholarly Works:

5. Bryant, Edwin F. The Yoga Sutras of Patanjali: A New Edition, Translation, and Commentary with Insights from the Traditional Commentators. New York: North Point Press, 2009.Comprehensive scholarly translation with extensive commentary drawing from classical sources
6. White, David Gordon. The Yoga Sutra of Patanjali: A Biography. Princeton: Princeton University Press, 2014.Historical and cultural analysis of the text's development and influence
7. Chapple, Christopher Key. Reading Patanjali Without Prejudice: New Translation of the Yoga Sutras with

Commentary. Delhi: D.K. Printworld, 2004.Academic translation with contemporary philosophical insights

8. Whicher, Ian. The Integrity of the Yoga Darsana: A Reconsideration of Classical Yoga. Albany: SUNY Press, 1998.Scholarly analysis of yoga philosophy and its internal coherence

9. Larson, Gerald James. Classical Samkhya: An Interpretation of Its History and Meaning. Delhi: Motilal Banarsidass, 1979.Essential background on Samkhya philosophy underlying the Yoga Sutras

Chapter 12: Integration of Patanjali Yoga Sutra in Daily Life

Practical Application Books:

1.DiNardo, Kelly, and Amy Pearce-Hayden. Living the Sutras: A Guide to Yoga Wisdom beyond the Mat. Boston: Shambhala Publications, 2018.Practical guide for applying yogic principles in contemporary life

2.Fendler, Susan. The Daily Guide to the Yoga Sutras: Bringing Ancient Wisdom to Modern Practice. Self-published, 2024.Daily applications and reflections on the sutras

3.Cope, Stephen. The Wisdom of Yoga: A Seeker's Guide to Extraordinary Living. New York: Bantam, 2006.Integration of yogic psychology with Western psychology

4.Lasater, Judith Hanson. Living Your Yoga: Finding the Spiritual in Everyday Life. Berkeley: Rodmell Press, 2000.Practical applications of yoga philosophy in daily living

5.Gates, Rolf. Meditations from the Mat: Daily Reflections on the Path of Yoga. New York: Anchor Books, 2002.Daily reflections connecting yoga philosophy to practical life

6.Stone, Michael. The Inner Tradition of Yoga: A Guide to Yoga Philosophy for the Contemporary Practitioner. Boston: Shambhala Publications, 2008.Modern interpretation of classical yoga philosophy

Academic and Research Articles

7.Jacobsen, Knut A. "The Institutionalization of the Ethics of 'Non-Harm' (Ahiṃsā) in Ancient India and Its Philosophical and Religious Significance." Journal of Ethics 16, no. 3 (2012): 287-309.

8.Burley, Mikel. "Classical Sāṃkhya and Yoga: An Indian Metaphysics of Experience." Routledge Studies in Asian Religion and Philosophy. London: Routledge, 2007.

9.Feuerstein, Georg. "The Philosophy of Classical Yoga." Inner Traditions International (1996).

10.Chapple, Christopher Key. "Yoga and the Path of the Urban Mystic." Journal of the American Academy of Religion 62, no. 4 (1994): 1031-1043.

Index

A

Absolute Freedom (Kaivalya Pada) · 113
Altered States of Consciousness · 10
Artificial Intelligence and Consciousness · 5
Asana (postures) · 115
Atman · 7

B

Biochemical Changes · 41
Biology of Belief · 63, 175
Biology of Stress · 73
Bliss Sheath · 16
Brahman · 7, 9, 10
Breaking the Addiction to the Past · v, 53, 175

C

Cellular Benefits of Meditation · 34
Cellular Renewal Meditation · 37, 39
Cognitive and Psychological Approaches · 4
Concentration (Samadhi Pada) · 113
Consciousness · 3, 4, 172, 173
Consciousness and Maya · 9
Consciousness and Reality · 11
Consciousness and the Cosmos · 3
Consciousness as a Bridge · 12
Consciousness as Fundamental · 8

Consciousness in Healthcare · 12
Consciousness in Hindu Philosophy · 6
Contemplation of Ishvara · 115
Contemplative Inquiry · 45
Core Meditation Traditions · 41
Creation as an Act of Consciousness · 11
Cultivating Positive Expectancy · v, 63, 64, 176

D

Development of Discriminative Discernment · 116
Dharana (concentration) · 115
Dhyana (meditation) · 115

E

Emotional Connection · v, 98, 178
Epigenetic Effects · 35
Epigenetics · 87, 88
Ethics · 12
Ethics and Consciousness · 12
Expectancy-Biology Loop · 64
Experiences (Vibhuti Pada) · 113

F

Focused Attention Meditation · 41
Food Sheath · 14
Free Will and Determinism · 11
Future of Mind-Body Medicine · v

G

Global Workspace Theory · 4

H

Heart Coherence Meditation · 101
HPA Axis · 31, 74

I

Inflammation · 19, 32, 34
Integration of Patanjali Yoga Sutra in Daily Life · 123
Intellectual Sheath · 15

L

Levels of Consciousness · 8
Living in the Quantum Field · v, 105, 178
Loving-Kindness Meditation · 21, 35, 43

M

Maya · 9
Meditation and Consciousness Exploration · 12
Meditation Bridge · 20
Meditation for Genetic Expression · v, 87, 177
Mental Sheath · 15
Mindfulness-Based Stress Reduction · 35, 44
Mitochondrial Function · 36

N

nature of reality · 3, 12
Neuroscientific Approaches · 4
Niyama (self-purification practices) · 114
Niyamas · 116, 119

O

Open Monitoring Meditation · 42
Oxidative Stress · 31, 34

P

Panpsychism · 5
Patanjali Yoga Sutra · 111
Placebo Effect · 16
Placebo Response Research · 67
Power of Meditation · v, 40, 174
Practice (Sadhana Pada) · 113
Pranayama (breath control) · 115
Pratyahara (sense withdrawal) · 115
Primacy of Consciousness · 9
Psychology · 172
Purpose and Meaning · 34

Q

Quantum Field Meditation · 66

R

Removal of Afflictions · 115

S

Samadhi (state of ecstatic union) · 115
Scientific and Hindu Views on Consciousness · 9
scientific study of consciousness · 4, 13
Self-Healing · v, 14, 173
Stilling the Modifications of the Mind · 115
Stress Response Pathways · 30, 74

T

Taittiriya Upanishad · 14
Telomerase · 19, 29, 77, 90, 92, 94, 99
Telomerase Solution · 19
Telomere Effect · xii, 19, 173
Telomeres · v, 18, 27, 28, 36, 38, 73, 74, 76, 174, 176
The Biochemistry of Belief · 17
The Eight Limbs of Yoga (Ashtanga Yoga) · 113
The Evolution of Consciousness · 11
The Hard Problem of Consciousness · 5, 10

The Limits of Knowledge · 12
The Mind-Body Problem · 11
The Nature of Self · 11
The Observer Effect · 10
The Panch Kosha Vivek · 14
The Practice of Kriya Yoga · 115
The Witness Consciousness · 8
Transcendental Meditation · 44

U

Unity of Consciousness · 10

V

Vital Air Sheath · 14
Viveka Khyati · 116

Y

Yama (ethical disciplines) · 114
Yamas · 119
Yoga and the Science of Consciousness · 9